T0285107

PRINCIPLES OF TRADITIONAL CHINESE MEDICINE

The Essential Guide to
Understanding the Human Body

XU XIANGCAI

YMAA Publication Center
Wolfeboro, NH USA

YMAA Publication Center
Main Office:
 PO Box 480
 Wolfeboro, New Hampshire, 03894
 800-668-8892 • info@ymaa.com • www.ymaa.com

20240627
Copyright ©2001 by Xu Xiangcai

ISBN 9781886969995 (print)
ISBN 9781594390975 (ebook)
ISBN 9781594394300 (hardcover)

Edited by Sharon Rose
Cover design by Richard Rossiter

Publisher's Cataloging in Publication
(Prepared by Quality Books Inc.)

Xu, Xiangcai.
 Principles of traditional Chinese medicine : the
essential guide to understanding the human body / Xu
 Xiangcai. — 1st ed.
 p. cm.
 Includes index.
 ISBN 1-886969-99-X

 1. Medicine, Chinese. 2. Qi gong. 3. Alternative
medicine. I. Title.

 R602. X89 2001   610.9'51
                            QBI1-2111

Disclaimer:
The authors and publisher of this material are NOT RESPONSIBLE in any
manner whatsoever for any injury which may occur through reading or following
the instructions in this manual.
The activities, physical or otherwise, described in this material may be too
strenuous or dangerous for some people, and the reader(s) should consult a
physician before engaging in them.

Printed in USA

Table of Contents

Chapter 5 Meridians, Channels and Collaterals

Chapter 6 Etiology and Occurrence of Disease

Chapter 7 Pathogenesis

Chapter 8 Diagnostic Method

Chapter 9 Differential Diagnosis and Treatment

Chapter 10 Preventative Therapeutic Principles

Glossary

Index

Foreword

I am delighted to learn that *Traditional Chinese Health Secrets* will soon come into the world. TCM has experienced many vicissitudes of times but has remained evergreen. It has made great contributions not only to the power and prosperity of our Chinese nation but to the enrichment and improvement of world medicine. Unfortunately, differences in nations, states and languages have slowed down its spreading and flowing outside China. Presently, however, an upsurge in learning, researching and applying Traditional Chinese Medicine (TCM) is unfolding. In order to bring the practice of TCM to all areas of the globe, Mr. Xu Xiangcai called intellectuals of noble aspirations and high intelligence together from Shandong and many other provinces in China to compile and translate this text. I believe that the day when the world's medicine is fully developed will be the day when TCM has spread throughout the world.

I am pleased to give it my recommendation.

Prof. Dr. Hu Ximing
*Deputy Minister of the Ministry of Public
Health of the People's Republic of China, Director
General of the State Administrative Bureau of
Traditional Chinese, Medicine and Pharmacology,
President of the World Federation of Acupuncture
Moxibustion Societies, Member of China
Association of Science & Technology, Deputy
President of All-China Association of Traditional
Chinese Medicine, President of China
Acupuncture & Moxibustion Society*

x

Foreword

The Chinese nation has been through a long, arduous course of struggling against diseases. Through this struggle, it has developed its own traditional medicine-Traditional Chinese Medicine and Pharmacology (TCMP), TCMP has a unique, comprehensive—both theories and clinical practice—scientific system including both theories and clinical practice.

Though its beginnings were several thousand years ago, the practice of TCM has been well preserved and continuously developed. TCM has special advantages, which include remarkable curative effects and few side effects. It is an effective means by which people can prevent and treat diseases and keep themselves strong and healthy. All achievements attained by any nation in the development of medicine are the public wealth of all mankind. They should not be confined within a single country. What is more, the need to set them free to flow throughout the world as quickly and precisely as possible is greater than that of any other kind of science. During my more than thirty years of being engaged in the practice of Traditional Chinese Medicine (TCM), I have been looking forward to the day when TCMP will have spread all over the world and made its contributions to the elimination of diseases of all mankind. However, it is to be deeply regretted that the pace of TCMP in extending outside China has been unsatisfactory due to the major difficulties involved in expressing its concepts in foreign languages.

Mr. Xu Xiangcai, a teacher of Shandong College of TCM, has sponsored and taken charge of the work of compilation and translation of such knowledge into English. This work is a great project, a large-scale scientific research, a courageous effort and a novel creation. I am deeply grateful to Mr. Xu Xiangcai and his compilers and translators, who have been working day and night for such a long time on this project. As a leader in the circles of TCM, I am duty-bound to do my best to support them.

I believe this text will be certain to find its position both in the history of Chinese medicine and in the history of world science and technology.

Mr. Zhang Qiwen
Member of the Standing Committee of All-China Association of TCM, Deputy Head of the Health Department of Shandong Province

Preface

Traditional Chinese Medicine (TCM) is one of China's great cultural heritages. Since the founding of the People's Republic of China in 1949, the treasure house of the theories of TCM has been continuously explored and the plentiful literature researched and compiled. The effort was guided by the farsighted TCM policy of the Chinese Communist Party and the Chinese government. As a result, great success has been achieved. Today, a worldwide upsurge has appeared in the studying and researching of TCM. To promote even more vigorous development of this trend in order that TCM may better serve all humankind, efforts are required to further it throughout the world. To bring this about, the language barriers must be overcome as soon as possible in order that TCM can be accurately expressed in foreign languages. Thus, the compilation and translation of a series of English-Chinese books of basic knowledge of TCM has become more urgent to serve the needs of medical and educational circles both inside and outside China.

In recent years, at the request of the health departments, satisfactory achievements have been made in researching the expression of TCM in English. Based on the investigation of the history and current state of the research work mentioned above, has been published to meet the needs of extending the knowledge of TCM around the world.

The encyclopedia consists of twenty-one volumes, each dealing with a particular branch of TCM. In the process of compilation, the distinguishing features of TCM have been given close attention and great efforts have been made to ensure that the content is scientific, practical, comprehensive and concise. The chief writers of the Chinese manuscripts include professors or associate professors with at least twenty years of practical clinical and/or teaching experience in TCM. The Chinese manuscript of each volume has been checked and approved by a specialist of the relevant branch of TCM. The team of the translators and revisers of the English versions consists of TCM specialists with a good command of English professional medical translators and teachers of English from TCM colleges or universities. At a symposium to standardize the English versions, scholars from twenty-two colleges and universities, research institutes of TCM, and other health institutes probed the question of how to express TCM in English more comprehensively, systematically and accurately. The English version of each volume was re-examined and then final checked. Obviously this encyclopedia will provide extensive reading material of TCM English for senior students in colleges of TCM in China and will also greatly benefit foreigners studying TCM. The responsible leaders of three organizations support the diligent efforts of compiling and translating this encyclopedia:

1. State Education Commission of the People's Republic of China

2. State Administrative Bureau of TCM and Pharmacy and the Education Commission

3. Health Department of Shandong Province

Under the direction of the Higher Education Department of the State Education Commission, the leading board of compilation and translation of this encyclopedia was created. The leaders of many colleges of TCM and pharmaceutical factories of TCM have also given assistance.

We hope that this encyclopedia will promote further and improve instruction of TCM in English at the colleges of TCM in China, cultivate the sharing of ideas of TCM in English in medical circles and give impetus to the study of TCM outside China.

CHAPTER 1

The Concept of Traditional Chinese Medicine

1.1 TRADITIONAL CHINESE MEDICINE (TCM)

Traditional Chinese Medicine is a discipline that deals with human physiology, pathology, diagnosis and the treatment and prevention of diseases. TCM encompasses a specific, integrated system of theory, which comes from a history of several thousand years of clinical experience. TCM develops from the experience of the Chinese people in their long struggle against diseases. As a result, TCM has contributed a great deal to the promotion of health and prosperity of the Chinese nation and to the further development of medical sciences all over the world as well.

1.2 THEORETICAL SYSTEM OF TCM

The theoretical system of TCM consists of the theories of *yin* and *yang*, the five elements, *zang-fu* organs, meridians, pathogenesis, syndrome and techniques of diagnosis. It also includes the therapeutic principles of health preservation and the six natural factors. It is a theoretical system much influenced by ancient materialism and dialectics, with the doctrine on *yin* and *yang* and the concept of integrated whole as its guiding principle. This concept is based in the physiology and pathology of the *zang-fu* organs and meridians. The diagnostic and therapeutic features of TCM include *bianzheng lunzhi*, which is a selection of treatment based on differential diagnosis.

1.3 CHARACTERISTIC FEATURES OF TCM

TCM is mainly characterized by its specific diagnostic techniques and therapeutic principles based on a practitioner's interpretation of the physiological functions and pathological changes of the human body. For instance, TCM regards the body as an integrated whole, closely interconnected by *zang-fu* organs, channels and collaterals that maintain a close link with the outer world. Where the development of disease is concerned, TCM stresses that endogenous pathogenic factors (namely, seven abnormal emotions) and exogenous pathogenic factors (namely, six exogenous pathogens) play an important role.

TCM utilizes four diagnostic techniques as its principal methods:

- Differentiation of diseases according to the theory of the *zan-fu* organs.
- Differential diagnosis according to the theory of the Six Channels.
- Differential diagnosis by the analysis of *wai*, *qi*, *ying* and *xue*.
- Differential diagnosis by the analysis of *san jiao* (tri-*jiao* or triple warmer/triple energizer).

TCM attaches great importance to the prevention and preventive treatment of disease. The practice of TCM maintains that the primary cause or root of a disease must be found and that a patient must be treated according to their physique as well as their seasonal and local conditions. In short, the characteristics of TCM can be summarized as:

- The concept of wholism.
- Selection of treatment based on differential diagnosis.

1.4 THE CONCEPT OF WHOLISM

The concept of wholism refers to a general view of the human body as a single, integrated entity that inter-relates with nature.

The human body is composed of a variety of tissues and organs and each of these performs a particular function and contributes to the life activities of the whole body. Thus, the human body is an integral whole, in that its constituent parts are inseparable in structure and connected with and conditioned by one another.

Because humankind exists in nature, the human body is affected directly or indirectly by any changes that occur in nature.

1.5 *BIANZHENG LUNZHI*

The word *bian* means comprehensive analysis and the word *zheng* refers to symptoms and signs. *Zheng*, however, not only refers to a mere combination of symptoms, but to a pathological generalization of a disease in a certain stage and the relation between body resistance and pathological agents.

When the two words are combined to form the word *bianzheng*, the term refers to the clinical data collected by the four diagnostic techniques of TCM: detection, analysis, summary and diagnosis. The patient's symptoms and signs are detected, analyzed and summarized thus establishing a diagnosis.

When the word *lunzhi* is added, it means that a proper therapeutic program is drawn up according to the diagnosis made.

The differential diagnosis known as *Bianzheng Lunzhi* is a fundamental principle of TCM that allows for the recognition and treatment of disease.

1.6 TREATMENT OF THE SAME DISEASE WITH DIFFERENT THERAPEUTIC METHODS

Disease that is in different stages may manifest itself by different syndromes and, therefore, can be treated with different therapeutic methods. Let us look at measles for example. In the early stage, when the appearance of the skin eruption is delayed and incomplete, the principle for promoting eruption must be applied. In its middle stage, when the lung-heat is the main syndrome, the practice of clearing away the lung-heat is indicated. Finally in the late stages, when lingering heat impairs *yin* in the lungs and stomach, the method of nourishing *yin* in order to clear away the lung-heat must be adopted.

1.7 TREATMENT OF DIFFERENT DISEASES WITH THE SAME THERAPY

The same therapy can be employed to treat different diseases that manifest themselves by the same syndrome. For example, both prolapse of rectum due to protracted illness and uterine prolapse can be treated by the therapy of elevating spleen-*qi* if the two ailments manifest themselves by sinking the *qi* of the middle-*jiao*.

CHAPTER 2

Yin-yang and the Five-element Theory

2.1 *YIN-YANG* DOCTRINE

According to ancient Chinese philosophy the *yin* and *yang* are two opposite categories. In the beginning, their meanings were quite simple, referring to turning away from or facing the sunlight respectively. Later, the *yin* and *yang* principles were used to describe an endless variety of things such as weather (cold or warm), position (downward or upward, right or left, internal or external), moving condition (mobile or static) and so on. The philosophers of ancient times observed that each phenomenon had two aspects, which were opposites regardless of the focus. Thus, the *yin* and *yang* theory is known as the basic law of the universe.

Yin and *yang* theory states that a natural phenomena contains two opposite aspects, thus forming the concept of the unity of opposites. Generally speaking, things active, external, upward, hot, bright, functional and hyperfunctional are of *yang* nature, while those that are static, internal, downward, cold, dark, substantial and hypofunctional are *yin* in nature.

Yin-yang doctrine is used to illustrate the sources and primary forms of movement of all things in the universe and the causes of their beginning and end.

As a theoretical tool in TCM, the *yin-yang* doctrine was applied to the study of physiology and pathology of the body and to diagnosis and treatment of diseases.

2.2 THE UNITY OF *YIN* AND *YANG* AS TWO OPPOSITES

Every thing and phenomenon in nature has two opposite aspects, *yin* and *yang*, which are manifested mainly in their mutual restraint and struggle. For example, the motions of celestial bodies, including the sun and the moon and the climactic changes of the four seasons, are the specific manifestations of the unity of opposites between *yin* and *yang*.

The Unity of Thoughts of Medicine and Book of Changes states that violent motion should be suppressed by tranquility, thus the hyperactivity of *yin* is restrained by *yang*. This implies that there is a relation of mutual restraint and mutual struggle between motion and tranquility. In other words, two mutually opposite aspects of anything always restrain one another through struggle.

When the *yin* and *yang* theory is applied to the body, the two opposites do not exist in a balanced state, rather they oppose each other. Through this kind of opposition and struggle a dynamic equilibrium can be established within the body. It is only through constant restraint and struggle that all things can develop and undergo change.

2.3 INTERDEPENDENCE BETWEEN *YIN* AND *YANG*

Although *yin* and *yang* are opposites and oppose each other, they are also interdependent. Without its opposite aspect, neither can exist independently, so each of the two opposite aspects is the condition for the other's existence. The chapter "Great Treatise on *Yin-Yang* Classification of Natural Phenomena" written by Su Wen states, "*Yin* is installed in the interior as the substantial basis of *yang*, while *yang* remains on the exterior as the manifestation of the function of *yin*." This statement best illustrates the relation of the interdependence between *yin* and *yang*. Here *yin* and *yang* refer to substance and function respectively. Substance exists within the body, while function manifests itself on the exterior of the body. *Yang* on the exterior is the manifestation of the activities of the substance within the body, while *yin* within the body serves as the substantial basis of functional activities. If each of the two opposite aspects cease to be the condition for the other's existence, no generation or growth is likely to occur.

2.4 WANE AND WAX OF *YIN* AND *YANG*

The opposition, mutual restraint, interdependence and interaction between *yin* and *yang* are not in a static or unchangeable condition. Rather they are constantly moving and changing. That is to say, within certain limits and during a certain period of time exists the alternation of the wane (decline) of *yin* followed by the wax (growth) of *yang* and vice versa. As an example we can look at the climate. From winter to spring and on to summer, the climate turns gradually from cold to warm to hot. This process is known as the wane of *yin* and wax of *yang* meaning that the winter cold gradually lessens as the heat of summer gradually increases. When summer turns from autumn to winter, the temperature turns from hot to cool and cold and thus is known as the wane of *yang* and wax of *yin*. In reference to the human body, *yang* is overabundant during the daytime. The *yang* is termed excitement while the *yin* is termed inhibition. After the middle of the night, *yang* begins to grow, at noon, *yang-qi* is excessive and the body's function turns gradually from being inhibited into being excited. Conversely, from noon until dusk, *yang-qi* wanes while *yin-qi* waxes and the body's physiological function turns from being excited to being inhibited. Therefore, the wane and wax of *yin* and *yang* help to maintain a dynamic equilibrium.

2.5 CLASSIFICATION OF THE STRUCTURES OF THE BODY IN TERMS OF *YIN* AND *YANG*

The unity of the human body can be understood as a relationship between two opposites. It is generally assumed that the upper part of the body, the surface, external sides, limbs and six *fu* organs pertain to *yang*, while the lower portion, interior, abdomen and five *zang* organs pertain to *yin*.

The equilibrium of *yin* and *yang* refers to the state of perfect harmony between *yin* and *yang*. Normal life activities of the body result from this harmonious relationship. This dynamic relationship is necessary for good health.

Relative Excessiveness of *Yin* or *Yang*. An excess of *yin* or *yang* beyond their normal levels promotes pathological changes. According to the principle of dynamic equilibrium between *yin* and *yang*, an excess of each of these two opposite aspects results in relative deficient other. Disease, according to TCM theory, results from an excess of *yin* or *yang* pathogens depending on what is deficient.

Excess *Yang*. When a *yang* pathogen is in excess it contributes to illness and inhibits *yin*. An excess of *yang* or *yang* pathogen is a pathological change resulting from *yang* excess beyond normal levels. It is stated in the *Da Lun* written by Su Wen, "An excess of *yang* produces heat syndrome." Excessive *yang* produces heat and thus gives rise to excessive heat syndrome.

Excess *Yin*. An excess of *yin* or *yin* pathogen is a pathological change resulting from *yin* in excess beyond normal levels. As is stated in the *Da Lun*, "An excess of *yin* leads to disorder of *yang* and produces cold syndrome." Thus, an excess of *yin* causes cold syndrome of the excess type.

Insufficient *Yin* or *Yang*. Insufficient *yin* or *yang* is a pathological change in which either *yin* or *yang* is below normal levels. According to the principle of dynamic equilibrium between *yin* and *yang*, deficient either leads to hyperactivity of the other. The main contradiction of diseases due to insufficient *yin* or *yang* lies in deficient *yin*-essence or *yang-qi*.

Deficient *Yang*. Deficient *yang* is unable to restrain *yin*, thus leading to hyperactivity of *yin* and cold syndrome of insufficiency type.

Insufficient *Yin*. When *yin* is deficient, it is unable to restrain *yang*, leading to relative hyperactivity of *yang* and heat syndrome. Thus, deficient *yin* is said to bring about heat syndrome of a weak type.

Deficient *Yang* Affecting *Yin* and Deficient *Yin* Affecting *Yang*. Deficient *yang* directly affects *yin*. When the *yang-qi* of the body is too weak to promote the production of *yin* fluid, insufficient *yin* results. Conversely, when the *yin* fluid of the body is too weak to promote the production of *yang-qi*, the result is insufficient *yang*.

Reestablishment of *Yang* from *Yin* and Reestablishment of *Yin* from *Yang*. As a method for treating *yang* deficiency syndrome, *yang*-invigorating herbs, food or drugs should be administered in combination with *yin*-nourishing drugs so as to promote the production of *yang-qi*.

As a method for treating *yin* deficiency syndrome, *yin*-nourishing herbs, food, or drugs should be administered accompanied by *yang*-invigorating remedies, so as to promote the production of *yin* fluid.

2.6 CLASSIFICATION OF DRUGS IN TERMS OF *YIN* AND *YANG*

In the practice of TCM, medicinal substances are differentiated in four ways:

- Nature
- Odor
- Taste
- Action

Properties of Medicinal Substances . Properties of medicinal substances refer mainly to their four pharmacological features, namely: cold, hot, warm, and cool. Among them, cold and cool are *yin* in nature, while warm and hot are *yang*. Remedies that can relieve or clear away the hot-syndrome are cold or cool nature, while those that can relieve or clear away cold syndrome are hot or warm in nature.

Five Tastes. TCM recognizes five different tastes, namely, acrid, sweet, sour, bitter, and salty. (TCM also recognized the absence of taste: bland.) Among them, acrid, sweet, and bland tastes belong to *yang*, while sour, bitter, and salty tastes to *yin*.

Remedies of the body are classified according to the tendency of their actions; remedies lift, lower, float, or sink. Among them, lifting and floating belong to *yang*, whereas lowering and sinking to *yin*. Remedies that produce the effects of elevating *yang*—inducing diaphoresis, dispelling wind, expelling cold, inducing vomiting, and resuscitation—act upward and outward. Their mechanisms of action are lifting and floating. On the other hand, those that are used for purgation, clearing away heat, inducing diuresis, tranquilization, suppressing *yin* and stopping wind, promoting digestion and relieving dyspepsia, lowering adverse flow of *qi* and astringency act downward and inward. Their mechanisms of action are lowering and sinking.

Clinically, to correct the imbalance of *yin* and *yang*, appropriate remedies are selected in accordance with their nature, depending upon excessiveness or deficient *yin* and *yang* in a disease.

2.7 FIVE-ELEMENT THEORY

The ancient Chinese found that in nature there exists a universal phenomenon that they called the five-element theory. The five-element doctrine was once used as a theoretical tool by ancient scholars to illustrate the nature of things, as well as the relationship between them on the bases of the properties, movements, and interactions of these five kinds of substances. In TCM, the five-element theory is chiefly used to explain the properties of viscera of the human body, their mutual relations, and their pathological changes.

Generation of the Five Elements. The five elements consist of wood, fire, earth, metal, and water. It was theorized that these elements generate each other. Wood generates fire, fire generates earth, earth generates metal, metal generates water, and water generates wood.

Degeneration of the Five Elements. Based on universal phenomena it was found that the elements also inhibit or restrict each other as well. Wood restricts earth, earth restricts water, water restricts fire, fire restricts metal, and metal restricts wood.

Interaction between the Five Elements. The five elements can over-restrict or reverse-restrict each other as well. As an example of over-restriction, wood can restrict earth, which results in insufficient earth.

As an example of reverse-restriction, wood should be restricted by metal; however, when wood is excessively strong it is not restricted by metal, rather it restricts metal.

Each of the five elements can be described by their properties as well.

The properties of the five elements are as follows:
- Wood has the property of free growth and unfolding.
- Fire has the property of warmth and flaring up.
- Earth has the property of generation, transformation, and receipt.

- Metal has the property of purification, descent, and astringency.
- Water has the property of nourishing and flowing downwards.

The five-element doctrine illustrates the connections existing between all things by the relationships among the five elements. It holds that nothing is in an isolated or static state; that is, everything is—or strives to be—in a state of harmonious balance maintained by the constant motion of intergeneration and inter-restriction. This is the basic premise of the five-element doctrine and it also serves as the foundation for dialectical materialism in ancient China.

2.8 REINFORCEMENT OF THE MOTHER-ORGAN IN THE CASE OF DEFICIENCY SYNDROME

Another therapeutic principle for treating deficiency syndrome is based on the concept of the mother-child relationship of intergeneration of the five elements.

The principle applied primarily to deficiency syndrome with mother-child relationship. For instance, consider the syndrome known as "water failing to nourish wood." In this situation, the liver (wood) is suffering from deficiency syndrome due to inability of the kidneys (water) to nourish the liver. To remedy the situation and restore balance, the kidneys, not the liver, are to be nourished. The reason: the kidneys are water and thus promote the liver, which is wood. This makes the kidneys the "mother organ" of the liver.

The mother-organ principle also holds true for acupuncture. In the treatment of deficiency syndrome of the child-organ, points pertaining to the mother-channel or mother-points are needled, reinforcing manipulation. For instance, in the case of a deficiency syndrome of the liver, *yingu* (a point on the kidney channel) is needled. In this sense, the disease of the child-organ is said to be eradicated by reinforcing the mother-organ.

2.9 REDUCTION OF THE CHILD-ORGAN IN THE CASE OF EXCESS SYNDROME

This is a therapeutic principle for treating the excess syndrome, based on the theory of the mother-child relationship of inter-generation of the five elements.

The principle is applied mainly to excess syndrome with mother-child relationship. For instance, excess syndrome demonstrated by an exuberance of the liver-fire can be treated by purging the fire of the heart (child-organ of the liver). This works because purgation of the heart-fire helps to reduce the liver-fire. In acupuncture, in the case of an excess syndrome of the mother organ, points pertaining to the child-channel are needled with purging manipulation. For instance, in the treatment of excess syndrome of the liver, either *shaofu* (H8, a point of the heart channel) or *xin jian* (Liv2, the child-point of the liver channel) is needled. In this sense, the disease of the mother-organ is cured by purging the child-organ.

2.10 A METHOD OF PROVIDING WATER FOR THE GROWTH OF WOOD

Here water refers to the kidneys, while wood to the liver. This is a method of restoring the liver (wood) -*yin* by nourishing the kidney (water) -*yin*, which is indicated for the relief of deficient liver-*yin* due to consumption of kidney-*yin*. It is also known as a method of nourishing the kidneys and the liver.

2.11 PROMOTE FIRE TO REINFORCE EARTH

The fire in the five elements originally and usually represents the heart of the five *zang* organs. However, there is another doctrine that states that the fire of *mingmen* (gate of life) warms the whole body. To benefit fire to reinforce, earth, fire refers to the fire from *mingmen*, i.e., kidney-*yang*. Earth corresponds to the spleen. This is a method of warming kidney-*yang* to invigorate spleen-*yang*, which is indicated in hypofunction of spleen-*yang* due to decline of kidney-*yang*.

2.12 MUTUAL PROMOTION OF METAL AND WATER

This is a method of reinforcing or nourishing the lungs (metal) and the kidneys (water) simultaneously in order to promote each other based on their mother-child relationship. In this instance, deficient lungs causes a failure of the lungs to distribute fluid to nourish the kidneys— or insufficient kidney-*yin* causes a failure of the kidneys to nourish the lungs—leading to deficient lung-*yin* and kidney-*yin*.

2.13 SUPPLEMENT METAL BY BUILDING EARTH

This is a method of replenishing and restoring the lung (metal) -*qi* by invigorating the spleen (earth) and replenishing *qi*. It is indicated in deficient lungs and spleen caused by failure of the spleen and stomach to nourish the lungs.

2.14 WARM EARTH TO RESTRAIN WATER

Here earth refers to the spleen and water to the kidneys. This is a method of treating retention of water within the body by warming spleen-*yang* or warming the kidneys to invigorate the spleen. It is usually used to treat edema and distention resulting from the overflow of pathogenic water dampness due to dysfunction of the spleen. If retention of water within the body is caused by failure of kidney-*yang* to warm spleen-*yang*, priority must be given to warming the kidneys, supplemented by invigorating the spleen.

2.15 INHIBIT WOOD TO SUPPORT EARTH

Here wood and earth refer to the liver and spleen, respectively. Inhibiting Wood to Support Earth is a method of treating hyperfunction of the liver and insufficient spleen by soothing the liver and invigorating the spleen. The concept: disperse the stagnated liver-*qi*, calm the liver to normalize stomach-*qi* or coordinate between the liver and spleen. It is indicated for the relief of hyperactivity of the liver (wood), which over-restricts the spleen (earth).

2.16 ASSIST METAL TO SUBDUE HYPERACTIVITY OF WOOD

Here metal and wood represent the lungs and liver, respectively. This method checks hyperactivity of the liver by purifying lung-*qi*; it is demonstrated by an exuberance of the liver-fire caused by the failure of lung-*qi* to keep pure and to descend.

2.17 PURGE THE HEART-FIRE (SOUTH) TO NOURISH THE KIDNEY-WATER (NORTH)

This therapy nourishes the kidney-water (located in the North) by purging the heart-fire (located in the South). It is indicated by excessive heart-fire and a breakdown of the normal physiological coordination between the heart and kidneys and is caused by insufficient kidney-*yin*. As the kidneys are an organ responsible for both water and fire, deficient kidney-*yin* may also give rise to over abundant ministerial fire, which differs from the heart-fire according to the five-element doctrine.

CHAPTER 3

Qi, Blood and Body Fluid

3.1 *Qi*

TCM holds that the term *qi* refers to the essential substance that creates the human body and maintains its life activities. Because *qi* has the properties of powerful vigor and constant movement and because it controls important physiological functions for the human body, TCM often explains the body's life activities in terms of the movement and change of *qi*.

The physiological functions of *qi* include
- Impulsing
- Warming
- Defending
- Communicating
- Regulating

Zhang Jingyue said. "The life of a human being relies totally upon *qi*."

Formation of *Qi*. The *qi* in the human body derives from the integration of three kinds of *qi*:
- Congenital *qi* inherited from the parents.
- Qi from food essence.
- Fresh air inhaled from the external atmosphere through the comprehensive action of the lungs, spleen, stomach, kidneys, and other *zang-fu* organs.

The formation of *qi* is closely related to the physiological functions of the kidneys, spleen, stomach, and lungs, as well as to genetic predisposition, diet, and natural environment. Among them the transporting-transforming function of the spleen and stomach is particularly important, for human placenta depends on the spleen and stomach to absorb nourishment as to maintain life activities. Meanwhile, the congenital essence-*qi* also relies on essential substances from food for replenishment.

Impulsing Function of *Qi*. *Qi*, as a vigorous essential substance, serves at least four vital roles:

- To promote and activate the body's growth and development.
- To promote and activate the physiological activities of various *zang-fu* organs, channels and collaterals.
- To produce and circulate blood.
- To form, distribute, and excrete body fluids.

Warming Function of *Qi*. The book *Nanjing* says: "*Qi* is responsible for warming the body," which means that it is the source of body heat. Only through the warming action of *qi* can the body's temperature be kept constant; can all *zang-fu* organs, channels, and collaterals and other structures perform their respective physiological functions; and can such liquid substances as blood and body fluids carry on regular circulation. "Blood flows in warm circumstances but coagulates in cold."

Defending Function of *Qi*. The defense mechanism of the body against disease is very complicated and involves the coordinated action of *qi*, blood, body fluids and *zang-fu* organs, channels, collaterals, and other structures. The defensive function of *qi* is reflected mainly in protecting the body surface against external pathogens.

Controlling Function of *Qi*. The controlling function of *qi* refers chiefly to the action of *qi* in reserving liquid substances, such as blood and body fluids. This includes keeping the blood flowing within the vessels so as to control the amount of the secretion and excretion of sweat, urine, saliva, stomach fluid, intestinal fluid, and semen and prevent their wasteful consumption.

Transforming Function of *Qi*. Transforming function implies various forms of conversions due to the movement of *qi*—namely, metabolism and transformation of the essence, *qi*, blood, or body fluids. For instance, the essence derived from food and drink transforms into *qi*, blood, and body fluids. The body fluids after being metabolized convert into sweat and urine, and the residues of food after digestion and absorption are turned into feces. All of these processes are manifestations of *qi*'s transforming action.

Primordial *Qi*. Primordial *qi* is also called "original *qi*." It is the primary motivational force for the human body's life activities and also the most essential substance for maintaining vital functions. The primordial *qi* is responsible for promoting the body's growth and development and for warming and activating all *zang-fu* organs, channels, collaterals, and other structures. It is formed from kidney-essence but depends on food essence transported by the spleen and stomach for nourishment and replenishment. It flows throughout the body via tri-*jiao*. "Tri-*jiao* is the passageway for the primordial *qi*."

Pectoral-*qi*. Pectoral-*qi* is composed of fresh air the lungs and the refined essence of food conveyed by the spleen combined in the *tan zhong* (thorax).

Pectoral-*qi* performs two main functions:

1. It acts on the respiratory tract to complete the breathing process and its vicissitudes bear relation to the strength of speech, voice, and respiration.

2. It runs through the vessels into the heart to keep *qi*-blood circulating. Therefore, the flow of *qi*-blood, the temperature and motility of the trunk and limbs, the perceptibility of visual and aural sensations, the strength and rhythm of the heartbeat, and so on, are all related to the vicissitudes of the pectoral-*qi*.

Since pectoral-*qi* accumulates in the thorax , the position of *xuli* (corresponding to the location where cardiac apex beats) is usually used to detect the vicissitudes of the pectoral-*qi*.

***Qi* of the Middle-*jiao*.** *Qi* of the middle-*jiao* refers to the functions of the spleen and stomach. Since the spleen is in charge of "sending up" and the stomach of "sending down," both are at the center of ascending-descending and exiting-entering movements of the body's *qi*. The ascending function of the spleen enables some internal organs of the body to keep themselves at their respective positions. Thus, sinking of *qi* of the middle-*jiao* may result in lassitude, loose stools, or protracted diarrhea with prolapse of rectum or even prolapse of internal organs.

Nutritive *Qi* (*Ying-qi*). Nutritive *qi* is a vital essence circulating with the blood in channels. The nutritive *qi*, as its name implies, is highly rich in nourishment and is mainly formed by the pure and pliable parts of the food essence transported by the spleen and stomach. It is distributed in the vessels as the component parts of blood. It has two physiological functions: It nourishes the whole body and it trans-forms into blood. In other words, the finest parts of essential substances from food constitute the major components of the nourishing *qi*. These components are nutrients necessary for the *zang-fu* organs, channels and collaterals, to carry on their physiological activities.

Defensive *Qi* (*Wei-qi*). Defensive *qi*, characterized by swiftness and toughness, like nutritive *qi*, is also derived from the essential substances of foods, but unlike nutritive *qi*, flows outside the vessels. Its physiolog-ical functions consist of three aspects:

1. It protects the body surface against exogenous pathogens.
2. It warms and nourishes the *zang-fu* organs, muscles, and skin with hairs.
3. It regulates and controls the opening and closing of pores for the discharge of sweat to maintain a relatively constant body temperature.
   The defensive *qi* is so named because of its protective action. By comparison, the nutritive *qi* belongs to *yin* and the defensive *qi* to *yang*, so they are also termed *ying-yin* (nutritive *yin*) and *wei-yang* (defensive *yang*), respectively.

Vital *Qi* (Genuine *Qi*). Vital *qi* permeates all parts of the body and consists of the congenital *qi* and the acquired *qi*. The chapter "Principles of Puncture and Relation Between Vital *Qi* and Pathogens" by Lingshu says: "The vital *qi* inherited from the parents, reproductive essence combines with the essential substances from food to fill the entire body." As opposed to pathogens, the vital *qi* is the healthy *qi* of the body.

Functioning of *Qi*. The movements of *qi* are called functioning of *qi*. Although the movements forms of *qi* are varied in form they can be summarized in four basic forms as follows: ascending, descending, outgoing, and incoming.

- Ascending action lifts *qi*.
- Descending action sinks *qi*.
- Outgoing action moves *qi* from an inner area to an outer area.
- Incoming action moves *qi* from an outer area to an inner area.

3.2 BLOOD

The blood is a red liquid substance rich in nutrients and circulates in the vessels. It is one of the essential substances that constitutes the human body and maintains the body's life activities. It possesses highly nourishing and moisturizing effects.

Formation of Blood. The nutritive *qi* and body fluids are regarded as the principal material basis for blood formation. Since they both are derived from food essence, the quality of the nutrients taken in and the functional state of the spleen and stomach directly influence the formation of blood. Moreover, food essence can also be transformed directly into blood.

Blood Serving Nutritive Function. Blood circulates continuously through the vessels and is carried to the *zang-fu* organs internally and to the skin, muscles, tendons, and bones externally. In this way, it exerts its fully nourishing and moisturizing effects on all of the organs and tissues of the body and thereby maintains its normal physiological activities. According to the *Nanjing*, "The blood is responsible for nourishing the body."

Blood As Material Basis for Mental Activities. To be full of vigor and to have perfect consciousness, keen perception, and free movement, the human body needs the blood for nourishment. For this reason, Su Wen states, "The blood is regarded as the material base of vitality of the human body and has to be nursed with caution."

Circulation of Blood. Normal circulation of the blood depends upon the coordination and balance between the propelling action and controlling action of *qi*. In the course of blood circulation, the heartbeat generates the flow of blood. Five important factors contribute to the circulation of blood:

- The lungs; dispersing-descending action.
- The convergence of vessels in the lungs.
- The control of normal *qi* flow by the liver.
- The spleen's function in keeping blood flowing within the vessels.
- The liver's ability to store blood.

In addition, blood temperature and unobstructed flow of *qi* through the vessels are closely related to circulation. The circulation of blood in the channels starts from the lung channel of hand-*taiyin* and ends at the liver channel of foot-*jueyin*, thus forming a circuit or a circle-like movement without terminal point.

3.3 BODY FLUID

Body fluid is a general term for all normal liquid components of the body, including the inner fluids existing in various organs and tissues, as well as their normal secretions, such as gastric juice, intestinal juice, saliva, and tears. Like *qi* and blood, body fluid is also an essential substance constituting the human body and contributing to the maintenance of its life activities.

Formation, Distribution, and Excretion of Body Fluid. A passage from the chapter "Another Exposition of Channel" by Su Wen says: "The nutritious part of a drink is absorbed in the stomach and then transported upward into the lungs by the spleen. Afterwards, it is dispersed to the whole body and partly sent down to the urinary bladder by the action of the lungs in regulating water metabolism and in so doing the body fluid extensively spreads out and flows in all channels." Thus one can see that

body fluid derived from food and drink is formed by:
- The stomach's preliminary digestion.
- The small intestine's separation of the refined substances.
- The spleen's role in transport.

The distribution and excretion of body fluid are accomplished by the joint action of many *zang-fu* organs, chiefly:
- The spleen's transportation.
- The lungs' dispersion and descent of the lungs.
- The warming-steaming and lifting clear-lowering turbid of the kidneys.

The body fluid uses the tri-*jiao* as its passageway for distribution and excretion.

Functions of the Body Fluid. Body fluid performs two functions: moistening and nourishing. When distributed throughout the body surface, it moistens the muscles and skin with hairs; when permeating through the body orifices, it moistens and protects eyes nose, mouth, and other openings. Additionally, when infiltrating into the vessels, it nourishes and smoothes the vessels and nourishes and moistens the internal organs. Finally, when seeping into the joint cavities, marrow cavities, and the skull, it lubricates the joints and nourishes and moistens the bone marrow, spinal cord, and brain.

3.4 RELATIONSHIP BETWEEN *QI*, BLOOD, AND BODY FLUIDS

***Qi* as the Commander of Blood.** As commander of blood, *qi* performs three main functions:
1. The production of blood
2. The propelling of blood
3. The control of blood circulation

"Production of blood" means that the formation of blood relies on the functional activities of *qi*. "Propelling of blood" means that *qi* is the motive force for blood flow. And, of course, the "control of blood circulation" indicates that the flow of blood within the vessels instead of extravasating depends mainly upon the dominant action of *qi*.

Blood as the Mother of *Qi*. The blood serves as the carrier of *qi*, supplying *qi* with adequate nutrients. Since *qi* is full of vigor and is easily lost, it must attach itself to both blood and body fluid. Thus blood is said to be "the mother of *qi*."

Body Fluid and Blood Is Derived from the Same Source. Both body fluid and blood are derived from food essence, hence they are said to have "a common source." Blood and body fluid usually influence each other. Therefore, for patients with excessive bleeding the practice of diaphoresis is not indicated. Additionally, for patients with deficient body fluid due to profuse sweating the treatment by removing blood stasis with drastic drugs is not indicated either. As is said in the chapter "Production and Convergence of Nutritive *Qi* and Defensive *Qi*" by Lingshu: "Diaphoresis is contraindicated in the case of consumption of blood and consumption of blood is contraindicated in the case of excessive sweating."

CHAPTER 4

Phase of Viscera

4.1 VISCERA

Zang (viscera) refers to internal organs of the body; *xiang* (phase or appearance) here refers mainly to the outward physiological and pathological manifestations. Zhang Jingyue, a famous physician in the Ming dynasty said in his *Classified Canon* (*Leijing*), "*zang* implies storage, while *xiang*, figure and appearance. Since viscera are located within the body and their phase is observed from the outside of the body, these two characters *zang* and *xiang* put together denote phase of viscera."

4.2 VISCERA-PHASE DOCTRINE

The viscera-phase doctrine states that by observing the physiological and pathological manifestations of the human body, one can study the physiological functions and pathological changes of its various viscera, their interactions and the interrelationship between visceral organs and structures of the body and the external environment.

Five *Zang* Organs. The heart, lungs, spleen, liver and kidneys are together known as the five *zang* organs. The *zang* organ was described in *The Yellow Emperor's Internal Canon of Medicine* (*Huangdi Neijing*) as an internal organ for storing and reserving. The common physiological property of the five *zang* organs is to produce and store vital essence.

Six *Fu* Organs. The gallbladder, stomach, small intestine, large intestine, urinary bladder, and tri-*jiao* (triple-burner or triple warmer) are known collectively as the six *fu* organs. The *fu* organ was referred to in the *Huangdi Neijing* as a container or a warehouse. The common functional property of the six *fu* organs is to take in, transport, and transform foodstuffs.

***Qiheng* (Extraordinary) *Fu* Organs.** The two characters, *qi* (this a different character than that of the character *qi* that means energy; this character has the same pinyin enunciation *qi*; here it means unusual) and *heng* (ordinary) put together imply "extraordinary."

Extraordinary *fu* organs, unlike ordinary ones, include the following six organs: brain, marrow, bone, vessel, gallbladder and uterus. Like the six *fu* organs morphologically, they are hollow in shape; like the *zang* organs functionally, they have the ability to store vital essence, but the inability to take in and transport foodstuffs. They are, therefore, called extraordinary *fu* organs.

4.3 THE HEART

The heart in TCM refers to both its anatomical entity and specific functions. The heart as an anatomical entity, located in the thorax above the diaphragm, is round at one end and a little sharp at another, just like an unopened lotus flower placed upside down and protected by the pericardium externally.

The heart governs the vessels and blood circulation and the mind takes *qi*-blood as its material basis. Therefore, the heart controls mental activities. In other words, it houses the mind. The heart, equivalent to the fire of the five elements, is thought to be the sunlight *yang* organ among the five *zang* organs; it coordinates the life activities of the whole body. The heart possesses two main functions:
- Control blood and vessels
- Regulate mental activities

The heart has its body opening in the tongue, its outward manifestations on the face, its particular emotion in joy, and its associated secretion in sweat. The heart and the small intestine have a exterior-interior relationship because of the interconnection of the heart channel of hand-*shaoyin* and the small intestine channel of hand-*taiyang*.

The Heart in Charge of Blood and Vessels. This heart performs two important functions: the maintenance of blood circulation and the control of vessel movement. The normal circulation of all of the blood in the vessel depends on the impulse of heart-*qi*; heart-*qi* transports the blood to all parts of the body for nutritive purposes. Repletion of heart-*qi* can maintain the normal strength, rate and rhythm of the heart. On the contrary, if heart-*qi* is insufficient, various cardiovascular diseases may ensue. The vessels, also called channels, are considered the house of blood; they are the passageways through which blood circulates.

The Heart in Charge of Mental Activities. This heart function is based on the premise that the heart houses the mind—the heart governs *shen*. The character *shen* has two meanings in TCM. In a broad sense, it is a general term for outward manifestations of life processes of the human body, commonly referred to as vitality. In a narrow sense, it refers to mental activities controlled by the heart, such as spirit, consciousness, and thinking. In modern physiology, all of these are thought of as the physiological functions of the cerebrum or its reflection of outward things.

The Heart Responsible for Joy. This aspect of the heart denotes that the physiological functions of the heart are related to joy, one of humankind's seven emotions. Literally, joy means happiness or pleasure. Usually, joy is a response to external favorable stimuli beneficial to the heart's ability to govern blood and vessels. As a result, the vessels are unblocked and *qi*-blood is harmonized. However, excessive joy tends to impair the functioning of the heart. As far as the heart's function of controlling mental activities is concerned, there are two kinds of pathological changes: hyperactivity and hypoactivity. Generally, the former gives rise to incessant laughter and the latter to sorrow.

The Heart Connects Vessels and Its Condition Is Reflected in Complexion. The TCM connection of the blood vessels to the heart implies that the movement of blood through the vessels is dominated by the heart. The heart has its outward manifestations on the face, which is extremely rich in blood vessels. Thus, the physiological functions of the heart can be detected through the changes in both color and luster on the face. Note the following conditions:

- When heart-*qi* is exuberant and the blood supply is sufficient, the complexion is rosy and lustrous.
- Insufficient heart-*qi* leads to pale and dark-turbid complexion.
- Deficient blood manifests a pallid complexion.
- Stagnation of the blood causes a darkish or purplish face.

Sweat Derived from Blood Regulated by the Heart. Sweat is a kind of body fluid discharged from pores under the steaming function of *yang-qi*. The discharge of sweat relies upon the opening-closing action of defensive *qi* on the striae of skin and muscles. When the striae are open, the sweat is let out; while they are closed, no sweating occurs. The sweat is transformed from body fluids and, furthermore, blood and body fluids are derived from food and drink. "Blood and sweat are from the same source." Blood is governed by the heart and sweat is said to be "the fluid of the heart."

The Heart with Its Specific Orifice in the Tongue. Heart-*qi* travels upward and reaches the tongue. Therefore it is believed that the heart opens into the tongue, which is said to be "the sprout of the heart." The tongue serves two main functions: it discriminates tastes and aids in speech, the performance of which depends on the heart's physiological functions in governing blood and vessels and in controlling mental activities. Moreover, the tongue is also richly supplied with blood vessels. Therefore, if the heart functions properly, the tongue must be ruddy, lustrous, soft, and nimble and its taste sensations must be keen and its speech fluent. On the contrary, if the heart fails to work properly, its physiological and pathological changes can also be reflected on the tongue. Consequently, the functional state of the heart can often be detected through observation of the tongue.

4.4 THE LUNGS

The lungs are situated in the thorax, one on each side. They are compared to the roof of a carriage due to their uppermost location among all of the *zang-fu* organs. They are also known as "delicate visceral organs" because their lobes are very delicate and tender, intolerant of cold and heat, and predisposed to invasion by pathogenic agents.

The lungs, equivalent to "metal" of the five elements, are the house of the soul and the dominator of *qi*. Their main jobs are to dominate *qi* and respiration, fulfill the dispersing and descending functions, participate in regulating water metabolism, and communicate with numerous vessels to achieve coordination of functional activities of the whole body. In this way, they assist the heart in maintaining normal circulation of *qi*-blood. The lungs, which extend upward toward the larynx and lead out through the nose, are related outward to the skin and its hairs. They are responsible for melancholy and have their associated secretion in nasal discharge. The lungs and the large intestine are related due to the interconnection of the lung channel of *hand-taiyin* and the large intestine channel of *hand-yangming*.

Qi and Respiration Dominated by the Lungs. The primary function of the lungs involves two aspects: the regulation of *qi* throughout the body and the control of respiration. The latter denotes that the lungs are visceral organs where interchange of *qi* inside and outside the body takes place, i.e., the exchange of gases between the body and its environment occurs through the breathing movements of the lungs. By continuously exhaling stale gas and inhaling fresh air instead, the lungs promote the formation of pectoral-*qi* and regulate the lifting-lowering and entering-exiting movements of *qi* and thereby maintain normal metabolism of the human body. This function is described in the chapter in the "Treatise on *Yin-Yang* Classification of Natural Phenomena" of the book by Su Wen: "The atmosphere communicates with the lungs."

Dispersing and Descending Functions of the Lungs. Literally, "dispersing" here means the upward diffusion and outward sending of lung-*qi* and the descending or lowering of lung-*qi* to keep the respiratory tract clean. The dispersing function of the lungs consists mainly in the following:

1. Discharging the stale gas from the body and its functional activities.

2. Distributing the food essence and body fluids transported by the spleen to all parts of the body and to the skin and its hairs externally.

3. Spreading defensive *qi* so as to control the open-and-close action of the striae of skin and muscles, thereby converting the metabolized body fluids into sweat to be removed from the body.

The descending function of the lungs, on the other hand, lies in:

1. Inspiring fresh air from the external environment.

2. Sending down the fresh air inspired and the body fluids as well as food essence transported from the spleen.

3. Purifying the foreign bodies in the lungs and the respiratory tract in order to keep the latter clean.

Water Metabolism Regulated by the Lungs. Water metabolism, here, refers to a physiological process by which body fluids are produced, distributed, and discharged. The lungs can regulate this process by maintaining normal flow, distribution and discharge of body fluids due to their dispersing and descending functions. Via their dispersing function, the lungs not only spread body fluids and food essence to all parts of body, they also control the discharge of sweat as well as the opening-closing action of the striae of skin and muscles. Via their descending function, the lungs send down fresh air into the kidneys. They also continuously send the part of the body fluids that was converted into urine to be excreted from the body via the kidneys and urinary bladder.

Convergence of Blood Vessels in the Lungs. The phrase, "convergence of blood vessels in the lungs" means that all blood flows along the vessels to all parts of the body through the lungs where the exchange of gases takes place. The circulation of blood relies upon the impulsion of *qi* and, with the lifting-lowering of *qi*, the blood flows to all parts of the body. Since the lungs control respiration and dominate the *qi* of the whole body, the circulation of blood depends to a certain extent on the spread and coordination of lung-*qi*.

The Lungs Are in Charge of Coordination of Functional Activities. This lung function may be summarized as follows:

1. The lungs make rhythmic breathing movements.
2. By means of their breathing movements, the lungs regulate the way that *qi* functions throughout the body (the lifting-lowering and entering-exiting movements of *qi*).
3. The lungs assist the heart in promoting and regulating blood circulation.
4. They help to maintain normal flow, distribution and discharge of body fluids.

The Lungs Are Responsible for Melancholy. Melancholy and sorrow as two modes of emotion, though slightly different from each other, exert roughly the same influence on physiological functions of the human body. Therefore, they both belong to the emotions of the lungs. After all, melancholy and sorrow are the emotional responses to unfavorable stimuli, bringing about a consuming effect on the *qi* of the body. As the lungs dominate *qi*, melancholy and sorrow are apt to impair the lungs. On the other hand, when the lungs are deficient, the body's tolerance to unfavorable stimuli is diminished and melancholy or sorrow is likely to occur.

The Lungs Connect with the Skin and Their Condition Is Reflected on Vellus Hairs. Here the skin and vellus hairs refer to the entire body surface including the skin, sweat glands, pili, etc. The skin with its hairs must be nourished by warmth and replenished moisture. These functions are accomplished by defensive *qi* and body fluids, respectively and thus form a protective barrier against external pathogens. Since the lungs dominate *qi* and perform the functions of dispersing outward defensive *qi* and sending the essence to the skin and vellus hairs, they are closely related to the skin and its hairs.

When the lungs function normally, the skin becomes compact and body resistance is enhanced. Otherwise, body resistance against foreign pathogens becomes weakened and such phenomena as hyperhidrosis and predisposition to common cold, wan, dry and lusterless skin and hairs, etc. are likely to occur. Conversely, the invasion of the skin and its hairs by foreign pathogenic agents causes closure of the striae of the skin and muscles. This results in the stagnation of defensive *qi*, frequently followed by failure of lung-*qi* to disperse and descend, which, in turn, leads to such pathological changes as occlusion of the striae of skin and muscles, stagnation of defensive *qi* and so on.

Nasal Discharge Derived from the Lungs. Nasal discharge is the mucuos secreted from mucous membrane of the nose, which moisten the nasal passage. The nose is the orifice of the lungs, and, under normal circumstances, its discharge moistens nasal lining instead of running out. In the case of an attack of the lungs by pathogenic cold, the lucid nasal discharge flows from the nose; in the case of an attack by heat, the nasal discharge becomes yellowish and thick; and in the case of an invasion by dryness, the nasal cavity becomes dry.

The Nose as the Window of the Lungs. The nose connects with the larynx and the larynx with the lungs; the nose and larynx are the passageway of respiration. "The nose is the external orifice of the lungs. The larynx is the gateway of the lungs."

Lung-*qi* governs both the sense of smell and the pronunciation in the larynx. Sound lung-*qi* with smooth breathing is accompanied by a keen sense of smell and sonorous voice. If foreign pathogens invade the lungs and come mostly from the nose and larynx, such symptoms as stuffy nose, running nose, sneezing, itching of the throat, and hoarseness may occur.

4.5 THE SPLEEN

The spleen is located in the middle-*jiao* (or middle warmer) below the diaphragm.

Its main physiological functions are:
- To transport, transform, and send up the nutrient.
- To keep the blood flowing in the vessel.

It is a chief visceral organ of the digestive system, upon the physiological functions of which the body's digestive activities depend. The nutrients transported and transformed by the spleen and stomach are used for production of *qi*-blood and body fluids, as well as for maintenance of the body's life activities. The spleen and stomach as "the source of *qi*-blood" are also known as "the material basis of the acquired constitution."

The spleen, which opens into the mouth and has its outward manifestations on the lips, corresponds to earth according to the theory of the five elements. It has its specific emotion in anxiety and its associated secretion in saliva. It also nourishes the muscles and limbs. In addition, the spleen and the stomach are exteriorly-interiorly related due to interconnecting of the spleen channel of foot-*taiyin* and the stomach channel of foot-*yangming*.

The Spleen Is in Charge of Transportation and Transformation. This function of the spleen involves digestion of food and drink and absorption and transportation of nutrients. The phrase "transporting-transforming action of the spleen on food" means that food in the stomach is digested and its nutrients are absorbed and then distributed to all parts of the body. If the spleen functions normally, the organism can obtain adequate nutrients to maintain its normal functioning. Conversely, if the spleen fails to transport and transform, normal digestion and absorption of food does not take place; instead a morbid condition occurs and is marked by abdominal distension, diarrhea, poor appetite, lassitude, emaciation, or even other symptoms due to insufficient *qi*-blood supply.

"The transporting-transforming action of the spleen on water" means the spleen's function of absorbing, conveying, and spreading body fluids. That is to say, the spleen transports the fluids absorbed from food and drink to the lungs to be distributed to all parts of the body, thereby fulfilling its nourishing-moistening role. The surplus fluids are turned into sweat and urine to be removed from the body under the functioning of the lungs and kidneys. Thus, normal function of the spleen in this respect can prevent body fluids from accumulating and such pathological changes as dampness, phlegm, and water-retention from occurring. On the contrary, dysfunction of the spleen in transporting-transforming fluids promotes fluid retention, development of the pathological changes mentioned above and even to edema.

The Spleen Is in Charge of Sending up Essential Substances. This function of the spleen refers to all processes concerned with the absorption of nutrients from food and drink and their upward transport to the heart, lungs, head, and eyes. In the meantime, these nutrients are transformed into *qi*-blood to nourish the whole body by the action of the heart and lungs.

The ability to send nutrients upward is the functional feature of the spleen. When this function of the spleen is carried out properly, the nutrients from food and drink can be absorbed and conveyed normally. In this way, plenty of vital *qi* eventually fills the body with vigor and vitality.

In addition, normal spleen function keeps the internal organs in their fixed positions. If the spleen fails to regularly transport-transform nutrients from food and thus fails to supply *qi*-blood, symptoms such as listlessness, weakness, dizziness, abdominal distension, and loose stool develop. If the spleen fails to lift spleen-*qi* and sinks it instead, pathological changes such as prolapse of the rectum due to protracted diarrhea—or even prolapse of other internal viscera—may occur.

Blood Flow Controlled by the Spleen. This function of the spleen refers to the spleen's capacity to keep the blood flowing within vessels.

The main mechanism of the spleen's control of blood flow is attributable to the commanding action of spleen-*qi* on blood circulation and is closely related to its capacity as the source of growth and development of *qi*-blood. If the spleen fails to transport and transform as needed, *qi*-blood becomes insufficient and its commanding action weakens, thereby producing various kinds of chronic hemorrhage.

The Spleen Is Responsible for Anxiety. Anxiety is considered the emotion of the spleen. However, it is also concerned with the function of the heart in controlling mental activities. Moderate anxiety does not exert any unfavorable influence on physiological functions of the organism; however, excessive anxiety may disturb the proper function of the spleen, thus resulting in such pathological manifestations as stagnation and depression of *qi*. If *qi* is depressed in the middle-*jiao* due to excessive anxiety, such symptoms as anorexia, epigastric stuffiness and distress, dizziness, etc., are likely to occur because the spleen is unable to properly transport, transform, and send up nutrients.

The Spleen Is Related to the Muscles. The development and strength of the muscles of the body are related to the function of the spleen and stomach in transport. As the spleen and stomach are the source of growth and development of *qi*-blood, the muscles in the whole body rely on the supply of nutrients from food transported by the spleen and stomach, whereby they are rendered well-developed and strong. If the spleen and stomach fail to function properly, the muscles become emaciated, weak and even paralyzed.

Saliva Derived from the Spleen. Saliva is a clear, watery fluid in the mouth. Its functions are:

- To moisten the oral cavity
- To protect the mucous membrane of the mouth
- To help to swallow and digest food

In the case of a lack of coordination between the spleen and stomach, saliva increases rapidly and profusely and spontaneous salivation ensues as a consequence. For this reason, saliva is referred to as the secretion of the spleen.

The Spleen's Body Opening is the Mouth and Its Outward Manifestations Are the Lips. The oral cavity is the uppermost end of the digestive tract. The spleen opens in the mouth, indicating that appetite and taste are closely related to the transportation and transformation functions of the spleen. When the spleen and stomach function properly in transport, taste and appetite is normal. On the contrary, dysfunction of the spleen in transport may cause abnormal tastes, such as tastelessness or sweet taste with sticky sensation in the mouth, thereby causing poor appetite.

The color and luster of the lips depend on the adequate supply of *qi*-blood transported by the spleen. Therefore, the spleen's functional state is reflected in the lips' color and luster.

4.6 THE LIVER

The liver is situated in the right hypochondriac region below the diaphragm in the abdomen. It is the house of mood, the storehouse of blood, and the controller of tendons. It corresponds to wood in the five elements and is characterized by ascending-spreading movement.

Its main physiological functions include the control of normal flow of *qi* and the storage of blood. It opens into the eyes and controls the tendons with its outward manifestations reflected on the nails. It has its specific emotion in anger and its associated secretion in tears. Moreover, the liver and gallbladder are exteriorly-interiorly related due to interconnecting of the liver channel of foot-*jueyin* and the gallbladder channel of foot-*shaoyang*.

Normal Flow of *Qi* Governed by the Liver. The liver is a solid visceral organ responsible for ascending-spreading movement, which is regarded as the physiological basis for its control of the normal flow of *qi*. This function of the liver is an important link in the regulatory functional activities of *qi* and promoting circulation of blood and body fluids. The liver governs normal flow of *qi* in a threefold action.

1. It regulates functional activities of *qi*, which refers to the lifting-lowering and entering-exiting movements of the liver. When the liver functions properly in this respect, *qi* and *qi*-blood function normally, channels flow freely, and the *zang-fu* organs and other structures perform normally. Conversely, dysfunction of the liver may manifest itself by two kinds of morbid conditions: hyperactivity and hypoactivity. In the case of hyperactivity of the liver, the following pathological changes may occur:

   • Upward adverse flow of liver-*qi*, characterized by distending pain of head and eyes, flushed face with congested eyes, irritability, restlessness, and so on.

   • Upward overflow of blood due to adverse flow of *qi*, marked by hemoptysis and even sudden syncope with unconsciousness.

   In the case of hypoactivity, the functioning of *qi* is impeded and may cause mental depression, distending pain in the chest, hypochondrium, breasts, or lower abdomen, etc.

2. The liver promotes the transporting-transforming function of the spleen and stomach. When the liver functions properly, it governs a normal flow of *qi* and greatly influences the lifting-lowering function of the spleen and stomach. For instance, dysfunction of the liver can impair the function of the spleen and stomach in lifting clear *qi* and lowering turbid *qi*. This dysfunction results in symptoms attributed to an attack of the spleen or stomach by the hyperactive liver-*qi*. Since bile is the aggregation of the surplus liver-essence, when the liver functions normally, it promotes the regular secretion and excretion of bile. Stagnation of liver-*qi* promotes irregular secretion and excretion of the bile and further impairs the function of the spleen and stomach in transportation and transformation.

3. The liver adjusts emotional activities. Whereas the heart primarily dominates emotional activities, the liver also closely relates to the activities of emotions. A normally functioning liver leads to normal functional *qi* activities, harmony of *qi*-blood, and proper functioning of the five *zang* organs, thus resulting in normal emotional activities. Conversely, hypofunction of the liver may lead to depression of liver-*qi*, manifested as a tendency toward melancholy and gloominess from even slight stimulation; hyperfunction of the liver results in adverse ascension of *yang-qi* and manifests as restlessness and irascibility after a slight stimulation. Repeated or persistent emotional abnormality, in turn, impairs the function of the liver and results in morbid changes such as stagnation of liver-*qi* or hyperactivity of liver-*yang*.

The Liver Stores Blood. This function is concerned with the liver's capability to store blood and regulate the volume of circulating blood. First, a certain amount of blood stored in the liver can restrain liver-*yang* from rising excessively. If the liver fails to function properly in storing blood, pathological changes such as deficient liver-blood or bleeding ensues. When liver-blood is not adequate enough to nourish the eyes, dryness and discomfort of the eyes with blurred vision or night blindness is likely to occur. If liver-blood fails to nourish the tendons, numbness of limbs and inflexible joints appears; if liver-blood is unable to replenish the reservoir of blood, scanty menstruation or even amenorrhea may occur in women. To sum up, the failure of the liver to store blood may give rise to such symptoms as menorrhagia or even metrorrhagia and metrostaxis.

Regulating the volume of blood circulating in the body is the principal role the liver plays. Under normal conditions, the volume of

circulating blood in every part of the body, especially the extremities, remains relatively constant but varies based on:
- The amount of activities in which the body engages
- Emotional changes
- Climactic changes, etc.

During strenuous activity or intense excitement, the liver releases stored blood to the peripheral portion of the body to meet its demands; during states of rest and calmness some of the circulating blood returns to the liver to be stored. In this case, the reduced activity of the body requires a relatively diminished demand for the peripheral blood.

Mood originates from the mind. Only when the liver functions properly in storing blood, can it house the mood properly. If the liver suffers a shortage of blood, the liver will be unable to control mood, and symptoms such as dreaminess with a tendency to be frightened, insomnia with restlessness, somnanbulism, somniloquy, etc., ensue.

The Liver Is Responsible for Anger. Anger is an emotional response of the human body to an unfavorable stimulation. With regard to its action on ability of the *qi* of the body to function properly, anger can make *yang-qi*, and hence *qi*-blood, ascend adversely. Since the normal flow of *qi* and the ascension of *yang-qi* are governed and promoted respectively by the liver, anger is referred to as the emotion of the liver. On the one hand, rage can cause excessive ascension of liver-*yang* and result in illness. "Excessive anger impairs the liver." On the other hand, deficient liver-*yin* or liver-blood in conjunction with hyperactivity of liver-*yang* leads to irascibility after a slight stimulation.

The Liver Related to Tendons with Its Outward Manifestations on the Nails. The tendons, attached to the bones and aggregating around the joints, join muscles to the joints. The tendons rely upon the liver for blood supply. Replete liver-blood nourishes the tendons, which, in turn, make the body move actively and nimbly. On the contrary, insufficient *qi*-blood of the liver leads to failure of the tendons to obtain sufficient nutrients and thus brings about such symptoms as tremors of hand and foot, numbness of limbs, difficulty in extension and flexion, convulsion, and so on.

The nails of both hands and feet are actually an extension of the tendons, so they are spoken of as "the remainders of the tendons." The amount of liver-blood directly affects the property and appearance of the nails. For example, sufficient liver-blood leads to tough and sturdy nails with ruddiness and luster. Conversely, insufficient liver-blood results in thin and frail nails with pallor dryness and without luster—and even deformed or cracked nails.

Tears Are the Secretion Derived from the Liver. Tears come from the eyes, which are the specific body openings of the liver. Therefore, tears are derived from the liver. Tears moisten and protect the eyes. Under normal physiological conditions, the lacrimal secretion just performs a moistening action inside the eyes but do not cause tears. Once a foreign object enters the eye, tears develop to clean the eyes and get rid of the foreign object. Under pathological conditions, however, abnormal secretion of the tears may occur. For instance, deficient liver-*yin* or liver-blood leads to insufficient lacrimal secretion, resulting in dryness and uncomfortable feeling of the eyes, while the liver channel's damp-heat leads to increased secretion in the eyes, epiphora induced by the wind, etc. Additionally, extreme grief can also greatly increase lacrimal secretion.

The Liver Has Its Specific Body Opening in the Eyes. As the liver channel connects upward with the ocular connectors and vision depends on the normal flow of liver-*qi* and the nutritive function of liver-blood, the liver is said "to open into the eyes." In addition, the essence and *qi* of the five *zang* organs and six *fu* organs all flow upward into the eyes, so an intrinsic relationship exists between the eyes and the *zang-fu* organs.

Owing to the extremely close relationship between the liver and the eyes, the former's functional state is usually reflected on the latter. For example, inadequacy of liver-*yin* or liver-blood leads to dryness and uncomfortable feeling of the eyes, blurred vision, or night blindness; wind-heat in the liver channel promotes conjunctival congestion and itching and pain in the eye and flaming-up of the liver-fire leads to conjunctivitis with nebula. Additionally, hyperactivity of liver-*yang* results in dizziness with dim eyesight and an "up-stirring" of the liver brings strabismus or squinting upward, etc.

4.7 THE KIDNEYS

The kidneys are situated in the waist, one on either side of the spinal column. They store the congenital essence, which is considered as the origin of *yin-yang* of *zang-fu* organs and the source of life of the human body. Hence, they are called "the origin of congenital constitution." They correspond to water according to the theory of the five elements.

The main functions of the kidneys are:
1. To store essence.
2. To dominate growth, development and reproduction.
3. To govern water metabolism and reception of air.

The kidneys produce marrow, which nourishes the bones. They have their outward manifestations on the hairs and their specific body openings in the ears and the two *yin*-orifices. They have their emotions in fear and fright and their associated secretion in spittle. The kidneys and the urinary bladder are exteriorly-interiorly related due to interconnecting of the kidney channel of foot-*shaoyin* and the urinary bladder channel of foot-*taiyang*.

Essence Stored by the Kidneys. This function of the kidneys refers to the storage of the kidneys' vital essence, which provides a favorable environment in which vital essence in the body can be brought into full play. In other words, plentiful essence is preserved without being unnecessarily eliminated so as to promote and maintain the body's growth, development, and reproduction.

As far as its source is concerned, the essence stored in the kidneys falls into two kinds: congenital essence and acquired essence. Congenital essence, inherited from the parents before birth, is the original substance that aids in the development of the embryo. Because of its function in reproducing offspring, it is also known as "reproductive essence." Acquired essence is transported and transformed by the spleen and stomach and is derived from food. Thus it is also named "food essence." Part of the food essence is supplied to aid the proper function of the *zang-fu* organs. The remainder of food essence is stored in the kidneys. Although the congenital essence and acquired essence do not have a common source, they are together stored in the kidneys, depending and reacting on each other. The congenital essence relies upon the acquired essence for a constant supply of nutrients, thereby smoothly performing its physiological functions. The acquired essence, in turn, depends upon the congenital essence for activation of its function of production and transformation.

Since the essence stored in the kidneys is the major material foundation for the body's growth, development, and reproduction, hypofunction of the kidneys in storing the essence leads to such symptoms as nocturnal emission and premature ejaculation and impaired normal growth, development, and reproduction of the body.

The Kidneys' Domination of Growth and Development. One of the chief physiological functions of kidney-essence is to promote the growth and development of the body. The chapter "Treatise on Innate Vital Essence in Ancient Times" by Su Wen clearly points out that the birth, growth, full development, senility and death of a human are closely related to the vicissitudes of kidney-essence. As the congenital essence is being continuously nourished and replenished by the acquired essence after birth, kidney-essence gradually becomes abundant, thereby giving rise to some physiological phenomena, such as growth of both permanent teeth and fine hairs during childhood. During the wax and wane of kidney-essence, the body goes through childhood to puberty, then to the prime of life, and finally old age. Throughout one's life, the growing conditions of the teeth, skeleton, and the hairs are important signs for vicissitudes of kidney-essence as well as for individuals of all ages.

Reproduction Dominated by the Kidneys. Reproduction is another main physiological function of kidney-essence. The reproductive power of the human body bears a close relation to kidney-essence. When the essence in the kidney is replenished to a certain degree during youth, the body produces a substance named *tian gui* (kidney-*yin*), which promotes the development and maturity of the sex glands. Then, a male begins to produce and ejaculate semen, while a female starts to have a regular menstruation with ovulation; that is to say, he or she possesses full reproductive power and is, therefore, said to reach puberty. After this, as the amount of kidney-essence decreases, the production of *tian gui* gradually slows until it is utterly consumed. The reproductive power also decreases accordingly until its complete loss due to gradual atrophy of the sex gland. Meanwhile, the person shifts from middle age to old age.

Water Metabolism Governed by the Kidneys. The metabolism of water is an important function of the kidneys. This function regulates the conveyance, distribution, and discharge of body fluids and maintains the balance of water metabolism within the body through the functioning of kidney-*qi*.

Metabolism of body fluids is achieved through ingestion of the stomach, transportation-transformation of the spleen, the dispersing and descending functions of the lungs, and steaming and ascending actions of the kidneys with tri-*jiao*. The tri-*jiao* acts as the water passage through which body fluids are transported to all parts of the body. The metabolized body fluids convert into sweat, urine, and gas to be eliminated from the body. The regulation of body fluids by the spleen, lungs and other viscera relies upon the steaming and ascending actions of kidney-*qi*; in short, steaming and ascending actions of kidney-*qi* govern metabolism of all body fluids. This is especially true of the formation and excretion of urine: these actions bear direct relation to the steaming and ascending actions of kidney-*qi*, and the formation and excretion of urine, in turn, play a very important role in maintaining the balance of water metabolism.

The Kidneys Govern the Reception of Air. The kidneys' control over the reception of air means that the kidneys control the normal exchange of gases between the body and its environment. In other words, although the lungs dominate the body's respiratory function, the body relies on the storing function of the kidneys to determine the release and exchange of gases. If the kidneys function normally, breathing is even, moderate and harmonious. Hypofunction of the kidneys, however, gives rise to a morbid condition marked by shallow breathing, prolonged exhalation, and shortened inhalation.

The Kidneys Are Responsible for Fear. Fear is a psychic reaction to something dreaded. It is similar to fright in implication, but fright is sudden while fear is anticipated. Both fright and fear are the emotions attributed to the kidneys. However, these emotions are in general related to the heart, which controls all mental activities (including emotions), and impairment of the heart-mind may bring about fear with cowardice.

The Kidneys Dominate Bones and their Physiological States Are Reflected on Hairs. The bones depend for their nourishment on the marrow, which is produced from kidney-essence. Therefore, the kidneys are said to be "in charge of the bones." The growth, development, and repair of the skeleton require the nourishment of kidney-essence.

- Abundance of kidney-essence leads to the plenitude of the bone marrow, resulting in a sturdy-robust skeleton and agile-powerful motions of the limbs.
- Deficient kidney-essence causes the depletion of bone marrow and debility of bones.

Because of the progressive decline of kidney-*qi* in elderly persons, their bones are adequately nourished by the bone marrow. Thus, elders often develop osteoporosis, a tendency of bones to fracture.

Similar to bone, teeth are nourished by kidney-essence. When kidney-essence is adequate, teeth are solid and unlikely to shed. Additionally, as the *yangming* channels of both hand and foot reach the teeth, some morbid conditions of the teeth are also related to those of the stomach and intestines.

The growth of hair completely relies on the supply of the kidney-essence and blood. The kidneys store the essence, so their condition may be reflected on the hairs. Since blood has the function of nourishing the hairs, the hairs are called "the remainder of blood." Generally speaking, premature senility, dry and withered hairs, premature gray hair, and hair loss are all related to insufficient kidney-essence or deficient blood.

Spittle Derived from Kidneys. Spittle is a thick fluid in the mouth. It is transformed from kidney-essence and then swallowed instead of being spit out. It has the function of moisturizing kidney-essence. Therefore, a great deal of spitting or long-standing spitting easily impairs kidney-essence. In addition, spittle also bears some relation to the spleen and stomach.

The Kidneys Have Their Openings in the Ears and Two *Yin*-Orifices. One's ability to hear depends upon whether kidney-essence is replete or not. For instance, repletion of kidney-essence promotes plenitude of the marrow and fullness of the brain and sharp and quick hearing follows as a result. Conversely, depletion of kidney-essence may results in tinnitus and even deafness. This is why the kidneys are said "to open into the ears."

The two *yin*-orifices refer to anterior *yin*-orifice and posterior *yin*-orifice, the former being the urethra and the latter, the anus.

Regarding the urethra. Urination is related to the function of the urinary bladder but depends on the functioning of kidney-*qi* for its accomplishment. Therefore, frequent urination is related to dysfunction of kidney-*qi*.

Regarding the anus. Defecation, although dependent upon the transportation of the large intestine, depends also on the normal function of kidney-*qi* as well. As examples, *Deficient kidney-*yin* may lead to constipation due to dryness of the intestinal juice. *Deficient kidney-*yang* promotes constipation or diarrhea due to disturbance in *qi* transformation and failure of the kidneys to store essence and control urination and defecation gives rise to protracted diarrhea or incontinence of feces.

The Gate of Life. The term gate of life was first found in "On the Root and Knot of Channel" by Lingshu, which states, "The gate of life is in the eye." However, the book *Nanjing* claimed that "There are the two kidneys in a human body, the left one being the kidney proper and the right the gate of life. The gate of life is the house of essence and mind and also the home of primordial *qi*. Since then, this thesis has attracted considerable attention of physicians, who advanced various opinions on the location and physiological functions of the gate of life. Now most scholars hold that fire from the gate of life is roughly equivalent to kidney-*yang* and the water from it to kidney-*yin*.

4.8 THE GALLBLADDER

Attached to the liver and located in between the hepatic lobes, the gallbladder is the first of the six *fu* organs. It is exteriorly-interiorly related to the liver because of the interconnection between their channels.

Because of the duality of its nature, the gallbladder is categorized as one of the six *fu* organs and as one of the extraordinary *fu* organs.

- Like the *fu* organs, it excretes bile to help digest food.

- Unlike ordinary *fu* organs, it does not receive and transport food and water. Instead, it stores "refined juice" or bile. In this sense, the gallbladder is described as belonging to the extraordinary *fu* organs.

The Gallbladder as a *Fu* Organ for Storing Refined Juice. "Storing refined juice" denotes that the gallbladder stores a pure fluid— or bile—that is bitter in taste and yellow-green in color, and that originates from the essence of liver-*qi*, converges into the gallbladder, and is excreted to the small intestine to help digestion. This functional activity of the gallbladder is an important basis for normal functioning of the spleen and stomach in transporting-transforming food.

The Gallbladder Stores and Excretes Bile. The main function of the gallbladder is to store and excrete bile, the production and excretion of which are controlled and regulated by the liver's control of *qi* flow. Consequently, if the liver functions properly, the gallbladder regularly and freely excretes bile and the spleen and stomach also normally conduct the transportation and transformation functions. When depression of liver-*qi* obstructs the excretion of bile, the following symptoms may appear: distending pain in the hypochondriac region, poor appetite, abdominal distension, loose stool, etc. If the bile flows upward, one may experience a bitter taste in the mouth and vomiting of yellow-green and bitter fluid. In the case of an overflow of the bile, jaundice may ensue.

4.9 THE STOMACH

The stomach, located in middle-*jiao* and also known as the gastric cavity, is divided into three parts: upper, middle, and lower. The upper part of the gastric cavity refers mainly to the cardia, its middle part to the body of stomach, and its lower part to the pylorus. The main function of the stomach is to receive and decompose food. The functional feature of stomach-*qi* is descending. The stomach is exteriorly-interiorly related to the spleen due to interconnection between their channels.

The Stomach Performs the Function of Receiving and Decomposing Food. The food mass coming from the mouth through the esophagus enters the stomach via the cardia and is received and contained by the stomach. Under the actions of stomach-*qi* and stomach-fluid, the food in the stomach is at first digested into chyme and is then carried into the small intestine to be further digested.

This function of the stomach is of great importance in maintaining the body's life activities and enhancing its resistance against disease; since food is the source for the production of *qi* –blood, it is the material basis for vital functions of the *zang-fu* organs. As mentioned in the chapter "On Pulses of Healthy People" by Su Wen, "Human depends for survival on food and water, without which human cannot live long."

The Stomach as the Reservoir of Food. Food passes from the mouth through the esophagus into the stomach, i.e., the stomach receives and contains all kinds of food. It is, therefore, also known as the "big barn" or "reservoir of food." As the *qi*-blood of the human body originates from food and drink, the stomach is also called "the reservoir of *qi*-blood from food." As stated by Ling Shu, "The vital *qi* existing within the human body comes from the food which is reserved and transformed in the stomach, so the stomach is regarded as the reservoir of *qi*-blood from food."

Descending Function of the Stomach. The descending function of the stomach, along with the ascending function of the spleen, comprises the functions of the whole digestive system of the body. In fact, the descending function of the stomach includes the activity of the small intestine to transfer the residues of food to the large intestine and that of the large intestine to turn the wastes into feces to be excreted from the body. The decomposed food in the stomach must move down to the small intestine to be first digested and absorbed. In this sense, sending food downward is a normal function of the stomach. In short, the regular descending action of the stomach is necessary to properly process food. So without the descent of stomach-*qi*, adverse rising of stomach-*qi* may occur, marked by belching with acid regurgitation, nausea, vomiting, hiccups, etc.

Stomach-*qi*. The term stomach-*qi* usually has two senses: narrow and broad. In a narrow sense, it refers only to the physiological functions of the stomach, particularly those of receiving and decomposing food. In a broad sense, however, it signifies the common physiological functions of both the spleen and stomach in receiving, digesting, transporting, and transforming food. Since the spleen and stomach are the source for the production of *qi*-blood, the vicissitudes of the body's *qi*-blood can be reflected in the pulse and a moderate and smooth pulse is referred to as "pulse with stomach-*qi*." Stomach-*qi* is of great importance in the human body. Clinically, doctors attach much importance to it, regarding it as an important principle of treatment.

4.10 THE SMALL INTESTINE

The small intestine is a long, tube-like organ in the abdomen, with its upper outlet connected by the pylorus with the lower outlet of the stomach and its lower outlet communicating with the upper outlet of the large intestine through the ileocecum. The main physiological functions of the small intestine are to temporarily store and further digest the partially digested food of the stomach and to separate the useful substances from the waste ones. The small intestine has a exterior-or-interior relation with the heart because of the interconnection between their channels.

The Small Intestine Stores and Digests Food. The function of the small intestine in storing has three basic implications. First, the small intestine receives the preliminarily digested food from the stomach. Secondly, it temporarily stores the food received there for a certain time in order to be further digested and absorbed. Finally, the small intestine further digests the food and converts it into refined nutritious substances.

The Small Intestine Separates the Useful Substances from the Waste. The chief function of the small intestine may be summarized in three aspects.
   1. The small intestine separates the digested food into two parts, the refined nutritious substances and the residues of the food.
   2. It absorbs the refined nutritious substances and transfers downward the residues of the food to the large intestine.
   3. It absorbs a considerable amount of fluid while absorbing the refined nutritious substances.

As a result of its ability to absorb fluid, the small intestine separates the refined nutritious substances from the waste ones, thereby promoting regular urination and defecation. Because this function of the small intestine is quite important in the process of forming the refined nutritious substances from food, it also furnishes an essential basis for the functioning of the spleen in sending up essential substances. For this reason, dysfunction of the small intestine may cause diarrhea resulting from "sinking of clear *qi*." This is known as "small intestine diarrhea," which is often treated by diuresis to dry the feces.

4.11 THE LARGE INTESTINE

The large intestine is situated in the abdomen, with its upper end connected to the small intestine by the ileocecum and its lower end being the anus. The main function of the large intestine is to convey and transform waste products. It is exteriorly-interiorly related with the lungs due to the interconnection between their channels.

The Large Intestine Conveys and Transforms Waste Products. The large intestine receives food residue sent down from the small intestine and, in the process of conveying them, absorbs a part of the surplus fluid and then turns it into feces to be eliminated from the body by the anus. Thus, it is stated in the chapter "Secret Classic in Emperor's Library" by Su Wen: "The large intestine is an organ for conveyance accompanied by formation of feces."

4.12 THE URINARY BLADDER

The urinary bladder, situated in the center of the lower abdomen, is an organ for storing and discharging urine. It communicates directly with the kidneys, to which it is exteriorly-interiorly related due to the interconnection between their channels.

Urinary Bladder Stores and Discharges Urine. The main function of the urinary bladder is to store and discharge urine. This function is accomplished through normal function of kidney-*qi*. Urine is formed from body fluids through the action of kidney-*qi* and is then sent to the urinary bladder, where part of it is retained and then automatically discharged from the body. A disorder of the urinary bladder usually manifests itself by frequency and urgency of urination, dribbling urination or incontinence of urine. These morbid conditions are mostly related to the dysfunction of kidney-*qi*.

4.13 THE TRI-*JIAO*

Tri-*jiao*, a general term for the upper, middle and lower *jiao* is regarded as one of the six *fu* organs. Early in Chinese history, the book, *Nanjing*, presented the view that "Tri-*jiao* exists merely nominally, it is not the entity of an organ." This *fu* organ aroused much controversy in later ages. However, it is now generally accepted that the main functions of tri-*jiao* are to pass (serve as a passageway for) various kinds of *qi* and to circulate body fluids. It is exteriorly-interiorly related to the pericardium. Since its functional activities are most extensively involved in the body covering its upper, middle and lower portions, it was once named "solitary *fu* organ."

Tri-*jiao* as a Passageway of Various Kinds of *Qi*. Tri-*jiao*, a passageway for ascending, descending, in-going and out-going *qi*, is the site of functional activity of *qi* within the body. Therefore, tri-*jiao* has the function of passing various kinds of *qi*. Primordial *qi*, the most essential *qi* of the body, must revitalize the whole body through tri-*jiao*. Therefore, a passage from the book *Nanjing* says:" Tri-*jiao* is the thoroughfare of primordial *qi* where the *qi* of the three portions of the body passes through the five *zang-* and six *fu* organs." To sum up, it is a passageway for ascending-descending and entering-exiting *qi*, which is actually distributed to five *zang* and six *fu* organs and further to all parts of the body through tri-*jiao*.

Tri-*jiao* as a Pathway for Circulation of Fluid. Su Wen states: "Tri-*jiao* is an organ in charge of water circulation where body fluids flow smoothly." It is thus clear that tri-*jiao* performs the function of dredging water passages, thereby serving as the pathway for lifting-lowering and entering-exiting of body fluids. Water metabolism is accomplished through the coordination of many viscera such as the lungs, spleen, stomach, intestines, kidneys, and urinary bladder, with tri-*jiao* as its passageway so that body fluids can ascend-descend and enter-exit normally. If the water passages, namely tri-*jiao*, are blocked, the distributive and regulative functions of the lungs, spleen, kidneys, and others are hard to fulfill.

The Upper-*jiao*. The upper-*jiao* refers mainly to the thorax above the diaphragm, including the heart, lungs and head. The upper limbs are sometimes also grouped into the upper-*jiao*. Its physiological function is to distribute the vital essence throughout the body. As pointed out in the chapter "Production and Convergence of Nutritive *Qi* and Defensive *Qi*" by Ling Shu: "The upper-*jiao* resembles a sprayer." That is to say, the upper-*jiao* is responsible for upward dispersion and outward spread of the nutrients and its functional state is compared to the natural fog-dew that permeates throughout the earth to nourish all things.

The Middle-*jiao*. The middle-*jiao* refers usually to the epigastrium below the diaphragm and above the umbilicus, including such viscera as the spleen, stomach, liver, and gallbladder. Its physiological functions are to digest food and to transport and transform the nutrients. "The middle-*jiao* resembles a fermentation vat," which "separates the useful substances from the waste and steams the essentials of food and water." Here the functions of the spleen and stomach—decomposing, transporting, and transforming food—are compared to a fermentative process.

The Lower-*jiao*. The lower-*jiao* refers generally to the lower portion of the body cavity below the stomach, consisting of the small intestine, large intestine, kidneys, urinary bladder, etc. Its physiological function is to excrete food residues and urine. The phrase, "lower-*jiao* resembling water passages" means that excretory function of the lower-*jiao* is similar to the drainage system in a city.

4.14 THE BRAIN

The brain is located in the cranium and is composed of converging marrow. The doctrine of visceral phase attributes the physiological functions and pathological changes of the brain to the heart and respectively to the five *zang* organs. The doctrine holds that "Like a king, the heart governs all of the vital functions of the body, including mental activities," and "as the dominator of the five *zang* organs and six *fu* organs, it houses the mind." In the meantime, the spirit, consciousness and thinking of the human body are connected with the five *zang* organs. For instance, the heart houses spirit and is in charge of joy; the liver houses mood and is in charge of anger; the spleen houses ideas and is in charge of anxiety; the lungs house the soul and are in charge of sorrow; and the kidneys house one's will and are in charge of fear. A passage from chapter "Great Puzzle" by Ling Shu says: "The vital essence of the five *zang* organs and six *fu* organs all flows up into the eyes and provides the material basis for visual function" and the ocular connectors "communicate with the brain." It is also said in the chapter "Oral Instruction" of the same chapter, "Insufficient vital essence of the head leads to the empty feeling in the brain, tinnitus, hung head with debility and vertigo." Thus, the morbid conditions of vision, hearing and mental state are related to the brain. During the Ming dynasty, the medical specialist Li Shizhen explicitly related the brain with mental activities, claiming that "The brain is the house of mental activities." Wang Ang of the Qing dynasty said: "The faculty of memory of the human body is derived from the brain." Afterward, Wang Qingren of the Qing dynasty attributed the functions of memory, vision, hearing, smell, speech, etc., to the brain on the basis of the predecessors' hypothesis.

4.15 MARROW

Marrow is classified into bone marrow, the spinal cord and the brain, all of which are manufactured by kidney-essence. The spinal cord connects upward with the brain, which is formed by the convergence of marrow. Therefore, the brain is called "the reservoir of marrow." In the case of exuberance of kidney-essence the reservoir of marrow" is replenished, the brain is well developed and the head completely fulfill its function as "house of intelligence." Conversely, in the case of deficient kidney-essence the "reservoir of marrow" fails to be nourished, hence resulting in a series of pathological changes. A passage from the chapter "Ling Lan Mi Dian" says: "The kidneys are responsible for staunchness of the body and intelligence of a person." In fact, this is the concrete manifestation of the function of the kidneys in dominating the bones and producing the marrow.

4.16 THE UTERUS

A woman's uterus or womb is situated in the lower abdomen posterior to the urinary bladder and is a reversed pear-shaped organ for menstruation and for creation of the fetus. Menstruation and pregnancy are both complex physiological courses in which *tian gui* (kidney-*yin*) plays the most important role. The *chong* and *ren* channels both originate from the uterus. In addition, the heart governs blood circulation, the liver stores blood, and the spleen keeps the blood flowing within the vessels, serving as the source of *qi*-blood. All are closely related to the uterus in physiological functions and pathological changes.

4.17 *TIAN GUI*

Tian gui is a kind of refined nutritious substance transformed from kidney-essence. It promotes and maintains the body's growth, development, and reproduction.

4.18 RELATIONSHIPS BETWEEN ORGANS

It is important to note important relationships between the various *zang-fu* organs.

Interior-Exterior Relationship between the Heart and the Small Intestine. The channels of the heart and the small intestine are interrelated to each other, so the heart and the small intestine are interiorly-exteriorly related. Pathologically, in the case of excessive fire in the heart, the heat may be transferred to the small intestine, resulting in oliguria, burning sensation during urination, pain during urination, etc. Conversely, the pathogenic heat of the small intestine may bring about flaring-up of the heart-fire along its own channel, manifested by dysphoria, crimson tongue, oral ulceration and so on.

Interior-Exterior Relationship between the Lungs and the Large Intestine. The channels of the lungs and the large intestine are interrelated to each other; therefore, the lungs and the large intestine are interiorly-exteriorly related. The purifying and descending functions of lung-*qi* help the large intestine to perform its transporting function. Likewise, proper function of the large intestine, in turn, aids lung-*qi* in fulfilling its purifying and descending functions. Pathologically, the lungs and the large intestine can affect each other. For example, the impairment of the purifying and descending functions of the lungs may give rise to difficulty in defecation and, conversely, the stagnation of large intestine-*qi* can impede the purifying and descending functions of lung-*qi*.

Interior-Exterior Relationship between the Spleen and the Stomach. Since the channels of the spleen and the stomach are interrelated to each other, the spleen and the stomach are interiorly-exteriorly related. The stomach dominates the receipt of food, while the spleen governs its transportation and transformation. The relationship between them may be summarized as follows: The spleen transports the nutrients for the stomach; both organs jointly accomplish the digestion of food and absorption and distribution of food essence that nourishes the entire body. Therefore, the spleen and the stomach "together provide a material basis for the acquired constitution." Spleen-*qi* tends to elevate while stomach-*qi* tends to lower, i.e., it is suitable for the spleen to send up and for the stomach to send down. The spleen corresponds to dampness and the stomach to dryness. Thus, the spleen is fit to be dried but is intolerant of dampness, and the stomach is fit to be moistened but is intolerant of dryness. Pathologically, hypofunction of the spleen due to dampness leads to failure to transport and elevate, thus impairing the functions of the stomach in receiving and lowering and there may appear poor appetite, nausea, epigastric distension, etc. On the contrary, the retention of food in the stomach due to intemperance of food intake promotes dysfunction of stomach-*qi* in descending and that of the spleen in elevating and transporting. In this case, symptoms such as abdominal distension, diarrhea, and others are likely to occur.

Interior-Exterior Relationship between the Liver and the Gallbladder. The channels of the liver and the gallbladder are interrelated to each other, so these two organs are interiorly-exteriorly related. The bile in the gallbladder is formed by the surplus of liver-essence. Furthermore, the storage and excretion of bile is closely connected to the liver's ability to control the normal flow of *qi*. If this function of the liver is abnormal, the secretion and excretion of bile is adversely affected. Conversely, obstructed excretion of bile may also impair the liver's ability to control the normal flow of *qi*.

Additionally, the liver and the gallbladder are also involved in mental activity, because the liver controls deliberation and the gallbladder governs judgment.

Interior-Exterior Relationship between the Kidneys and the Urinary Bladder. Because of the interrelation between the kidneys and the urinary bladder through their channels, they are interiorly-exteriorly related. The ability of the urinary bladder to store and excrete urine depends on the functioning of kidney-*qi*. When kidney-*qi* is sufficient, the kidneys adequately reserve *qi* and thus the urinary bladder opens and closes at the right moments. However, when kidney-*qi* is insufficient, disturbance in *qi* transformation occurs, and the kidneys fail to fulfill their reserving function and cause abnormal opening-closing of the urinary bladder. In this case, incontinence or frequent urination may occur.

Relationship between the Heart and the Lungs. The relationship between the heart and lungs embodies the interdependence and interaction between *qi* and blood. In short, the heart governs blood and blood circulation while the lungs dominate *qi* and respiration, and the link between them is created through the ability of pectoral-*qi* to connect the heart and the lungs and to promote breathing. Blood circulation and respiration can be enhanced by the coordination and balance of the two, and convergence of vessels in the lungs can aid the heart in maintaining blood circulation.

- Dysfunction of the lungs may lead to an abnormal flow or retardation of blood, manifested as an oppressive sensation in the chest, changes in heart rate or rhythm, bluish purple lips, or purplish tongue due to blood stasis.
- Deficient heart-*qi* and weakness of heart-*yang* may impair the lungs' ability to dominate *qi* and respiration due to an irregular flow of blood. The result is a morbid condition marked by coughing and rapid breathing.

Relationship between the Heart and the Spleen. The heart governs blood and the spleen keeps blood flowing within the vessels and provides *qi*-blood as the source of growth and development. Therefore, the relationship between the heart and the spleen is manifested chiefly in two aspects: the formation of blood and its circulation.

Regarding the formation of blood. The spleen's normal transportation function promotes normal blood cell growth, hence furnishing adequate blood supply for the heart. Regarding circulation. Vigorous spleen-*qi* guarantees the ability of the spleen to control blood flow within the vessels.

Pathologically, the heart and the spleen often influence each other. Consider the following:

- Excessive thinking gives rise both to internal consumption of heart-blood and to impairment of the spleen's ability to transport spleen-*qi*.
- Insufficient spleen-*qi* causes hypofunction of the spleen in growth and development and thus leads to deficient blood.
- This occurrence further weakens the heart's ability to govern blood.
- Additionally, the spleen's failure to keep the blood flowing within the vessels promotes the improper flow of blood as well as deficient heart-blood.

All of the above result in a morbid condition known as "deficient *qi* and blood in the heart and spleen" marked by palpitation, insomnia, dreaminess, anorexia, lassitude, and sallow complexion.

Relationship between the Heart and the Liver. Since the heart governs blood and the liver stores it, their relationship may be viewed from two aspects: blood circulation and mental activities.

Regarding blood circulation. Only when the heart promotes normal blood circulation can the liver store what it should store. Meanwhile, only when the liver adequately controls the normal flow of *qi* can the blood flow smoothly.

Regarding mental activities. The heart controls mental activities and the liver adjusts emotional activities. Therefore, the heart controls spirit, consciousness, thinking, and emotions, which are closely related to the liver's clearing function.

Pathologically, the inability of the liver to store blood leads to the heart's failure to govern blood, thus resulting in irregular blood flow. If extreme emotions produce pathogenic fire or further damage *yin*, the following morbid conditions may appear: excessive fire of both the heart and liver and deficient heart-*yin* and liver-*yin*.

Relationship between the Heart and the Kidneys. The heart corresponds to fire and is situated in the upper part of the body, while the kidneys correspond to water in the lower part of the body. Therefore, the relationship between the heart and kidneys is one of coordination and mutual assistance between fire and water. The heart-fire needs to go down to the kidneys while the kidney-water needs to go up to the heart. This is what is known as coordination between the heart and the kidneys or mutual assistance of fire and water. The discordance between water and fire may bring about a morbid condition known as "a breakdown of the balance between the heart and the kidneys." Insomnia, palpitation, dysphoria, lassitude in the loins and legs, nocturnal emission (in men), or coition while dreaming (in women) mark this condition. Furthermore, in the course of disease, the pathological interaction between the heart and kidneys is due to the close relationship between their respective *yin* and *yang*. For example, the water overflow due to insufficient kidney-*yang* can spread upward to the heart, manifested by edema, palpitation with fright, etc. This is what is called "impairment of the heart by retained fluid." On the other hand, deficient heart-*yin* can also involve kidney-*yin* below, thereby resulting in excessive fire due to *yin* deficiency.

Relationship between the Lungs and the Spleen. The relationship between the lungs and the spleen is chiefly manifested in two aspects: the formation of essence-*qi* and the metabolism of body fluids.

In the formation of essence-*qi*, the active functions include the respiratory function of the lungs and transporting-transforming function of the spleen. Fresh air (inhaled in the lungs) and food-essence (derived from the spleen and stomach) provide the primary basis for the formation of vital *qi* of the body. Therefore, the health of both the spleen and the lungs are necessary for healthy maintenance of vital *qi*.

In the metabolism of body fluids, the lungs' ability to disperse, descend, and maintain unobstructed water passages is beneficial to the spleen's transporting-transforming function. Conversely, the physiological activities of the spleen in transporting nutrients and fluids to the lungs are necessary for the lungs' ability to properly function in clearing and regulating water passages. In this respect, the spleen also provides the lungs with necessary nutrients.

As for pathological connections, insufficient spleen-*qi* usually promotes insufficient lung-*qi*. In other words, dysfunction of the spleen in transport leads to disorder of water metabolism and stagnancy of fluids, which then accumulates into phlegm and fluid-retention. These conditions impair the dispersing and descending functions of the lungs, resulting in a morbid condition marked by dyspnea and cough with copious sputum. "The spleen serves as the source of sputum and the lungs as its container."

The protracted lung-disease can also affect spleen-*qi*, accompanied by abdominal distension, poor appetite, loose stool, and so on.

Relationship between the Lungs and the Liver. The relationship between the lungs and the liver is mainly reflected in the regulation of functional activities of *qi*, because the lungs tend to sink *qi* and liver tends to lift it. For instance, excessive ascent of the liver or deficient descent of the lungs may lead to cough with dyspnea or even hemoptysis, a syndrome known as "the lungs attacked by excessive liver-fire." On the other hand, impairment of the lungs' ability to purify and descend combined with an overabundance of inner dryness or heat may also affect the liver. This results in stagnation of liver-*qi* and manifests as cramping pain and distension in the chest and hypochondrium, dizziness, headache, flushed face, and congested eyes.

Relationship between the Lungs and the Kidneys. The relationship between the lungs and the kidneys may be viewed mainly from two aspects: water metabolism and respiratory activities.

In regard to water metabolism, the lungs as "the upper source of fluid" rely upon kidney-*qi* for support. Conversely, the kidneys, which dominate metabolism of body fluids, also require support from the lungs (especially their ability to move *qi* downward and to clear water passages).

As for respiratory activities, the lungs govern the exchange of gases from air and the kidneys govern the reception of air. Therefore, sufficient kidney-*qi* helps the inhaled air sent down from the lungs be received in the kidneys. "The lungs are the dominator of *qi* and the kidneys its root."

As to pathological changes, impairment of the dispersing and descending function of the lungs and their failure to clear and regulate water passages adversely affects the kidneys and gives rise to oliguria and even edema. Similarly, if kidney-*qi* malfunctions, retained fluid may overflow upward, causing dyspnea or gasping cough with inability to lie flat. Either insufficient kidney-essence or deficient lungs with kidneys involved can bring about the kidneys' failure to receive air, marked by dyspnea on slight exertion and so on.

Since the lungs correspond to metal and the kidneys to water and since metal creates water according to the five-element theory, a relation of mutual promotion between lungs (metal) and kidneys (water) is inherent in their relationship. That is to say, lung-*yin* can replenish kidney-*yin* downward, which, in turn, can nourish lung-*yin* upward. Pathologically, deficient *yin* fluid of the lungs and that of the kidneys can frequently occur simultaneously, thereby causing the zygomatic regions to flush, e.g., hectic fever "like coming out from the bones," night sweats, dry cough with hoarseness, and lassitude in the loins and legs.

Relationship between the Liver and the Spleen. The liver stores blood and governs the normal flow of *qi*, while the spleen controls blood flow, dominates transportation and transformation, and serves as the source of generating *qi*-blood. The transporting-transforming function of the spleen is dependent on the clearing function of the liver, whose normal functioning, in turn, aids the spleen in transport.

Dysfunction of the liver—the inability to properly govern the normal flow of *qi*—may affect the spleen and result in a morbid condition called a lack of coordination between liver and spleen. Conversely, dysfunction of the spleen in transport may bring about the retention of damp-heat in the interior and further interfere with the function of the liver to maintain the unrestrained flow of *qi* and—with the excretion of bile—give rise to jaundice.

Moreover, there is a close relation between the liver and spleen as far as formation, storage, and circulation of blood are concerned. For instance, when the spleen functions well in transport and blood in abundance does not overflow, the liver has the proper amount of blood to store. Otherwise deficient liver-blood is likely to occur.

Relationship between the Liver and the Kidneys. Since the liver stores blood and the kidneys store *qi*-essence and since the blood and essence promote each other and transform themselves into each other, the liver and the kidneys form a close relationship with each other. In fact, they come from the same source. "*Yi* (the liver) and *Gui* (the kidneys) are from the same source. Therefore, essence and blood have a common source." Pathologically, they can affect each other, thus resulting in deficient essence and blood.

The liver governs normal flow of *qi* and the kidneys govern storage of essence. Thus, both restrain and oppose each other and yet complement each other. This interaction manifests as physiological functions such as menstruation and seminal emission. For this reason, disorder of either the liver or the kidneys may give rise to irregular menstruation in females and seminal emission without ejaculation in males.

There is also a mutual restraining and coordinating relation between *yin* and *yang* of both the liver and the kidneys. Deficiency or excess of one leads to excess or deficient other. For instance, deficient kidney-*yin* may bring about hyperactivity of liver-*yang* and result in a morbid condition called "water failing to nourish wood." Similarly, overabundance of the liver-fire may consume kidney-*yin*, giving rise to deficient kidney-*yin*. Additionally, both the liver and kidneys house the ministerial fire, the hyperactivity of which requires appropriate treatment for both organs.

Relationship between the Spleen and the Kidneys. The relationship between the spleen and kidneys consists primarily of two aspects: one refers to the influence on one's constitution and the other to the interaction of spleen and kidney functions.

Regarding constitutional makeup. The spleen governs the transportation and transformation of nutrients and is responsible for one's acquired constitution, and the kidneys are thought of as the root of *yin-yang* of the body and thus are responsible for one's congenital constitution. Physiologically, the spleen as the source of growth and development provides the material basis for the acquired constitution. Similarly, the kidneys store vital essence and energy and serve as the origin of congenital constitution.

The interaction between the two constitutions, embodied by the spleen and kidneys is illustrated below:

The production of *qi*-blood by the spleen depends on the warming-invigorating action of the kidneys, and, conversely, the transporting-transforming function of the spleen and the warming-invigorating action of kidney-*yang* influences the essence-*qi* stored in the kidneys.

Additionally, essence-*qi* also relies on the replenishment of *qi*-blood transformed from food. That is to say, the acquired nutrients are controlled by congenital essence-*qi* and supplied by innate essence-*qi*.

Regarding their functions. Aided by other *zang-fu* organs, the spleen and the kidneys coordinate their respective functions (in conveying fluid and dominating water) so as to maintain the balance in metabolism of body fluids.

Pathologically, the spleen and the kidneys influence and act upon each other. For example, congenital defect and weakness of the warming-invigorating action of the kidneys impairs the function of the spleen in generating *qi*-blood. Likewise, lack of proper care after birth and deficient *qi*-blood produced by the spleen leads to failure of the kidneys to store the essence from other *zang-fu* organs, which results in deficient kidney-essence.

In respect to transportation and transformation of food essence and water metabolism, failure of kidney-*yang* to warm and invigorate spleen-*yang* or protracted insufficient spleen-*yang* with the root of *yang-qi* involved may lead to insufficient *yang* of both the spleen and the kidneys.

CHAPTER 5

Meridians, Channels, and Collaterals

5.1 MERIDIAN DOCTRINE

The Meridian Doctrine, or the theory of channels and collaterals, deals with the physiological functions and the pathological changes of the system of the channels and collaterals and their relationship with the *zang-fu* organs.

5.2 CHANNELS AND COLLATERALS

Literally, the channel means the "route," and collateral, the "network." The channel is the cardinal conduit of the meridian system and the collateral is its branch. "Meridian" is the general term for both the channels and collaterals. The meridian system acts as specific passageways for the circulation of *qi* and blood throughout the body, the interconnection between visceral organs and extremities and the communication of the upper body with the lower and of the interior body parts with the exterior. The channels take a definite route, but the collaterals are widely distributed throughout the body like an interlacing network that combines all structures of the body such as the *zang-fu* organs, body orifices, skin, muscles, tendons, and bones into an integral whole.

5.3 MERIDIAN SYSTEM

The meridian system consists of the channels, collaterals, and their connective tissues. This system links the *zang-fu* organs internally and joins the tendons, muscles, and skin externally.

The channels may be classified into two categories: regular channels and extra channels. There are twelve regular channel: the three *yang* channels of hand and foot, as well as the three *yin* channels of both hand

and foot. The twelve regular channels are the main passages for the circulation of *qi* and blood.

There are eight extra channels: *du, ren, chong, dai, yingqiao, yangqiao, yinwei* and *Yangwei.* The eight extra channels perform the functions of governing, connecting and regulating the twelve regular channels.

The collaterals, which are the minor branches of the channels, are classified into three groups: major, superficial, and minute. The major collateral is the larger and main collateral of each channel. Each of the twelve regular channels as well as the *du* and *ren* channels possesses a major collateral, plus an extra large splenic collateral. They are known collectively as the fifteen major collaterals. The fifteen major collaterals can strengthen the relation between every two exteriorly-interiorly related channels on the body surface. The superficial collaterals are those that are located superficially and therefore often emerge on the skin. And the minute collaterals refer to all of the tiny collaterals.

The connective tissues of the meridian system involve the channel-musculatures and skin areas. They are the muscular system and the body surface, respectively, and they are distributed along the routes of the twelve regular channels.

5.4 TWELVE REGULAR CHANNELS

All of the names of the twelve regular channels are as follows:

> The lung channels of hand-*taiyin*
> The pericardium channel of hand-*jueyin*
> The heart channel of hand-*shaoyin*
> The large intestine channel of hand-*yangming*
> The tri-*jiao* channel of hand-*shaoyang*
> The small intestine channel of hand-*taiyang*
> The spleen channel of foot-*taiyin*
> The liver channel of foot-*jueyin*
> The kidney channel of foot-*shaoyin*
> The stomach channel of foot-*yangming*
> The gallbladder channel of foot-*shaoyang*
> The urinary bladder channel of foot-*taiyang*

Trends and Connections of Twelve Regular Channels. The orientation and connective law of the twelve regular channels is as follows:

- The three *yin* channels of the hand travel from the chest to the hands, connecting with the three *yang* channels of the hand at the ends of the fingers.

- The three *yang* channels of the hand travel from the ends of the fingers to the head, connecting with the three *yang* channels of the foot at the ends of the head and face.

- The three *yang* channels of the foot run from the head to the feet, connecting with the three *yin* channels of the foot at the ends of the toes.

- The three *yin* channels of the foot run from the feet to the abdomen, connecting with the three *yin* channels of the hand at the thoracic and abdominal cavities.

Distributive Law of Twelve Regular Channels. In the region of the upper and lower limbs, the three yin channels run along the medial aspect and the three yang channels along the lateral aspect. In general, the taiyin and yangming channels are located in the anterior, assuming the radial surface as the anterior part of the upper limbs and the tibial surface as the anterior part of the lower limbs. Likewise, the shaoyin and taiyang channels are located in the posterior part and the jueyin and shaoyang channels are on the middle line.

In the region of the head alone, *yangming* channels run on the face and forehead, *taiyang* channels on the cheek, vertex and *shaoyang* channels.

As to the trunk of the body, the three *yang* channels of the hand run in the scapular region.

Among the three *yang* channels of the foot, the *yangming* channel runs along the front of the body, the *taiyang* channel, along the posterior of the body and *shaoyang* channel, along the lateral body.

The three *yin* channels of the hand all come out from the axillae and the three *yin* channels of the foot go upward along the ventral aspect. Further, the order of the foot channels running along the ventral aspect from the medial to the lateral is *shaoyin, yangming, taiyin,* and then *jueyin.* Note: in reference to the medial sides of the two lower limbs, 8 cun above the medial malleoli, *jueyin* is located in the anterior, *taiyin* in the middle, and *shaoyin* in the posterior.

Exterior-Interior Relations of Twelve Regular Channels. The three *yin* and three *yang* channels of hand and foot are mutually linked by their branches and major collaterals. In this way, they form six pairs of exterior-interior relations. Among them, the *taiyang* channel and the *shaoyin* channel of the foot are related exteriorly-interiorly, as are the *shaoyang* and *jueyin* channels of the foot, and the *yangming* and *taiyin* channels of the foot. This is what is known as the "*yin-yang* of the foot."

Similarly, the *taiyang* and *shaoyin* channels of the hand are related exteriorly-interiorly, as are the *shaoyang* and the *jueyin* channels and the *yangming*, and the *taiyin* in channels of the hand. This is what is called the "*yin-yang* of the hand."

Order of Circulation of *Qi*-Blood in the Twelve Regular Channels. The twelve regular channels are distributed interiorly and exteriorly over the body. *Qi* and blood in the channels flow circularly in a definite order: from the lung channel of hand-*taiyin*, to the liver channel of foot-*jueyin*, and back to the lung channel in an endless way.

5.5 Eight Extra Channels

The eight extra channels include the *du, ren, chong, dai, yinqiao, yanqiao, yinwei,* and *yangwei* channels. Unlike the twelve regular channels, the eight extra channels are not regularly distributed, nor are they directly connected with *zang-fu* organs, The eight extra channels are not exteriorly-interiorly related to each other, either. That is why they are named as "extra" channels, distinct from the twelve regular ones.

The eight extra channels perform the following three functions:
- They strengthen the close relations between the twelve regular channels.
- They regulate *qi*-blood in the channels.
- They constitute the physiological and pathological media for connections between some *zang* organs, such as the liver and kidneys and the extraordinary *fu* organs, such as the uterus, brain and spinal cord.

***Du Mai* (*Du* Channel).** *Du* means governing and commanding. The *du* channel goes along the middle line of the back and frequently meets the three *yang* channels of both hand and foot and the *yangwei* channel. The *du* channel governs all of the *yang* channels of the entire body. That is why it is also named "The sea of the *yang* channels." Additionally, the *du* channel runs within the spinal column, ascends into the brain and divides into two branches pertaining separately to the two kidneys. As a result, it is closely concerned with the brain, spinal cord, and the kidneys.

Ren Mai (***Ren*** **Channel**). Literally the character *ren* means assuming or loading. The *ren* channel runs along the midline of the ventral side of the body and frequently meets the three *yin* channels of both hand and foot and the *yinwei* channel. The *ren* channel is loaded with the *qi*-blood of all of the *yin* channels of the body. Hence it is said to be "The sea of the *yin* channels."

The character *ren* also means pregnancy. The *ren* channel that arises from the uterus in women is related to conception.

Chong Mai (***Chong*** **Channel**). The Chinese character *chong* means thoroughfare. The *chong* channel ascends to the head and descends to the foot. It permeates throughout the whole body and serves as the communication center for the circulation of *qi*-blood. In fact, it can regulate the *qi*-blood of the twelve regular channels and is therefore said to be "The sea of the twelve regular channels."
The *chong* channel is also known as "The reservoir of blood" since it is closely related to menstruation in female.

Dai Mai (***Dai*** **Channel**). Literally, the character *dai* means belt. The *dai* channel originates from the hypochondriac region, runs obliquely downward through the *dai mai* point and then runs transversely around the waist like a belt. It can restrain all of the channels running vertically.

Yinwei Mai (***Yinwei*** **Channel**) **and** ***Yangwei*** **Mai (Yangwei Channel).** The character *wei* denotes connection. Thus, the *yinwei* channel connects all of the *yin* channels and *yangwei* channel connects all of the *yang* channels.

Yinqiao Mai (***Yinqiao*** **Channel**) **and** ***Yangqiao Mai*** (***Yangqiao*** **Channel).** The character *qiao* denotes agility. Originating from the heel, the *yinqiao* and *yangqiao* channels nourish the eyes and govern the opening and closing of the eyelids and the movement of the lower limbs. *Yinqiao* and *yangqiao* are in charge of the *yin* and *yang* of either side of the body respectively.

5.6 BRANCHES OF TWELVE REGULAR CHANNELS

The branches of the twelve regular channels originate respectively from the elbows and knees of the limbs at the point(s) through which the twelve regular channels pass. The branches of the twelve regular channels perform three physiological functions:

- They strengthen the inner connection between each pair of the exteriorly-interiorly-related channels.
- They promote the inner relation of the body proper because of their dominant action on the collaterals.
- They convey *qi*-blood to nourish the whole body.

5.7 *Fu Luo* (Superficial Collaterals)

The collaterals that are distributed on the body surface are named superficial collaterals. Described by Lingshu, they are "the shallow and often emergent collaterals."

5.8 *Sun Luo* (Minute Collaterals)

As is described in the chapter "Measurement of Channel" by Lingshu, "The little branches of the collaterals" are called minute collaterals. Thus, the tiny collaterals branching off from the big ones are named minute collaterals.

5.9 Twelve Skin Areas

Imagine the pattern that would emerge if one could really see the meridians on the surface of the skin. The sections of skin formed by this pattern make up the twelve skin areas. These skin areas are the sites where the *qi* of the twelve regular channels disperses.

The twelve skin areas assist in the treatment and diagnosis of disease. For instance, observing the morphological changes and discoloration on different skin areas helps to diagnose some disorders of the *zang-fu* organs and the meridians. Therefore, the application method—in this case, mild moxibustion and hot medicated compresses on certain areas of the skin—also helps to cure some morbid conditions of internal organs.

5.10 Twelve Channel-Musculatures

The channel-musculatures are the channels and collaterals where the muscular system is attached to each of the respective regular channels. The functions of the channel-musculatures rely on the nourishing action of *qi*-blood in the meridians and are coordinated by the twelve regular channels. Their main function is to bind the bones in order to make possible the flex-stretch movement of the body's joints.

5.11 PHYSIOLOGICAL FUNCTIONS OF MERIDIANS

The functional activities of the meridians are called channel-*qi*. The four primary physiological functions are:

- Connect all of the *zang-fu* organs with other structures and link the exterior with the interior and the upper with the lower.

- Circulate *qi*-blood to nourish the whole body.

- Play the inductive and conductive roles in pathological and therapeutic courses.

- Regulate the functional activities of the *zang-fu* organs.

CHAPTER 6

Etiology and Occurrence of Disease

6.1 DISEASE

A disease is commonly considered to be the outcome of the imbalance between *yin* and *yang*, organic trauma, and abnormality in physiological functions of the body. The concept of disease includes the following points:

- A disease is the outcome of pathogenic factors acting upon the body.
- It manifests itself as a life process of imbalance between *yin* and *yang*.
- It is a process undergoing constant changes, during which from beginning to end exists the struggle of opposites between impairment and repair and between obstruction and readjustment of the body.

6.2 OCCURRENCE OF DISEASE

The occurrence of a disease refers to the condition in which, under the action of some pathogenic factors, the human body loses the balance between *yin* and *yang*, its *zang-fu* organs are impaired, and its normal physiological functions are disturbed.

Humans are always affected by variations in weather and environmental factors. In the struggle to adapt and transform, humans maintain a relative balance between *yin* and *yang* within the body and its normal physiological functions. A disease may occur when radical or abnormal changes in natural environment go beyond the body's ability to readjust itself. Disease can also occur when the body cannot adapt to pathogens due to insufficient vital essence, thereby bringing about the imbalance between *yin* and *yang* and impairment of the *zang-fu* organs.

6.3 CAUSE OF DISEASE

The science dealing with the nature, characteristics, and laws of pathogenic factors and TCM reveals the cause of a disease not merely by means of visual observation, but, most importantly, by analysis of symptoms and signs on the basis of clinical manifestations of the disease. This procedure is known as tracing the cause of a disease by differentiation of symptoms and signs, which is a method of recognizing the cause of a disease characteristic of TCM.

All of the causes or conditions leading to imbalance between *yin* and *yang* in the body, impairment of the *zang-fu* organs, and abnormality in their physiological functions are known collectively as the cause of disease. For instance, disease can be caused by pathological products such as:

- The six climate conditions in excess (wind, cold, summer-heat, dampness, dryness, and fire)
- Epidemic pathogenic factors
- Impairment due to the seven emotions (joy, anger, melancholy, anxiety, grief, fear, and terror)
- Improper diet
- Overwork
- Various kinds of traumatic injuries
- Phlegm retention
- Blood stasis

6.4 THE THEORY OF THREE CATEGORIES OF ETIOLOGIC FACTORS

The Theory of Three Categories refers to the famous theory of etiologic taxonomy by Chen Yan of the Song dynasty in his book *Prescriptions Assigned to the Three Categories of Pathogenic Factors of Disease*. By combining pathogenic factors with the channels of the occurrence of disease, he developed the etiological classification of *xie* (pathogenic factor) into harmful *yin* and harmful *yang*. This theory was expanded upon in the *Neijing* and in *The Three Categories of Etiologic Factors Accounting for All Causes of Hundreds of Diseases* by Zhang Zhong Jing of the Han dynasty. The introduction of this theory, though far from perfect, gave an enormous impetus to the research into etiology in later ages.

The renowned theory proposes three categories of etiologic factors: exopathic, endopathic, and non-endo-exopathic. Specifically, exopathic causes of disease include six pathogenic factors (climates) invading the body from the outside, and endopathic causes include seven excessive emotions that directly damage internal organs. Non-endo-exopathic causes of disease include other pathogenic factors, such as improper diet, overwork, injuries caused by fall, knives and spears, and those caused by insects and animals.

6.5 *LIU YIN* (SIX CLIMATE CONDITIONS IN EXCESS AS PATHOGENIC FACTORS)

Lin yin is a general term for the six exopathic pathogenic factors; namely, wind, cold, summer-heat, dampness, dryness, and fire. *Yin* here means excess and overabundance—excess of one or more atmospheric influences that cause disease. Under normal circumstances the six different climactic conditions are necessary for the growth of all things on earth and, therefore, do no harm to the human body. However, these natural factors turn out to be pathogenic agents when:

- The six natural factors are excessive or deficient due to abnormal changes in weather.
- These factors change so rapidly that they exceed the body's resistance.
- Because of deficient its vital *qi*, the body's resistance declines too rapidly and is unable to adapt itself to the changes in weather.

6.6 CHARACTERISTICS OF SIX EXOPATHIC FACTORS

The following are characteristics of the six exopathic factors in excess:

1. When illness is caused by an excess of one or more the exopathic factors, the illness is commonly related to seasonal climates and the natural environment in which one lives. For example, diseases due to pathogenic wind occur more frequently in spring, and summer-heat disorders occur most often in summer. One is more likely to suffer from arthritis when living long in a damp place, and one will suffer from diseases due to dryness-heat and pathogenic fire when working in a hot environment.

2. Each of the six exogenous pathogenic factors can cause disease alone or more than two can do so simultaneously, e.g., wind, cold, and dampness combined as a pathogen cause stagnation-syndrome of *qi* and blood, common cold of wind-cold type and damp-heat diarrhea.

3. The exopathic factors not only interact in the course of a disease, but can also transform themselves into one another depending upon the conditions and nature of the disease's pathogenesis; syndromes change accordingly. For example, the pathogenic cold that invades the body from the exterior is liable to be transformed to heat due to the constitution of *yang* type, while chronic summer-dampness can be transformed to dryness and then impaired.

4. The exopathic factors cause disease through the following channels:
   * By way of superficial muscles
   * Through the mouth and nose
   * Through a combination of superficial muscles, the mouth and the nose

For instance, the cold-stroke syndrome of the *taiyang* channel is often caused by the entry of wind-cold pathogen, and an epidemic febrile disease is due chiefly to the invasion of pathogens via the mouth and nose.

The Wind Pathogen. Wind, prevailing in spring, exists all of the year round. Wind in excess and causing disease is known as pathogenic wind. The wind pathogen possesses the following features:

1. Characterized by upward and outgoing dispersion, it is *yang* in nature. As a pathogenic factor, wind usually promotes symptoms marked by perspiration. It may also invade the *yang* portion and often attacks the upper portion of the body, the *yang* channels, or superficial muscles.

2. Constant movement and rapid change characterize pathogenic wind. The fact that wind is in constant motion means migratory pain usually marks the disease. For instance, rheumatic fever causes the migratory pain in the joints, which is thus known as wind arthritis.

   Similarly, the fact that the wind pathogen changes rapidly causes diseases characterized by abrupt onset and variable changes. For example, German measles is marked by migratory itches on the skin and a change in the appearance of the skin.

3. Pathogenic wind is the predominant pathogenic factor. As the first one of the six exogenic pathogenic agents, wind is the predisposing factor contributing to exopathic diseases while all of the other pathogenic factors (cold, dampness, dryness) usually invade the human body in association with wind pathogen.

The Cold Pathogen. Cold, though prevalent in winter, is also very common in other seasons. Cold in excess and causing disease is referred to as pathogenic cold, which possesses the following characteristic features:

1. Pathogenic cold is liable to impair *yang-qi*. It is a manifestation of excessive *yin-qi*, which leads to disorder of *yang*. The restraint of the skin's function by the cold pathogen oppresses the defensive *yang*, manifesting itself as extreme cold and high fever. Likewise, a direct attack of pathogenic cold on the spleen and stomach impairs their *yang-qi* and thus results in abdominal pain and diarrhea.

2. Sometimes an invasion by pathogenic cold promotes retardation of the circulation of *qi* and blood in the body and blocks channels and collaterals. This causes a stagnation of a cold nature from which pain results. Often rheumatic arthritis appears, manifested by the symptoms of severe pain in the joints and aversion to cold.

3. An attack of pathogenic cold that results in a disturbance of the visceral function, closure of sweat pores, and contraction of muscles is attributed to contraction due to cold. This condition manifests in the body as muscles spasms.

The Summer-Heat Pathogen. Summer-heat exists only in summer and results from fire. Summer-heat in excess and causing disease is known as pathogenic summer-heat. Diseases produced by summer-heat display the following characteristics:

1. As a pathogenic agent that is *yang* in nature, summer-heat presents a series of *yang* heat symptoms, such as high fever, vexation, flushed face, rapid and racing pulse, etc.

2. The upward flow and dispersion of summer-heat pathogens lead to consumption of *qi* and body fluid. Invasion of summer-heat pathogens often causes excessive sweating due to the opening of sweat pores, which, in turn, leads to consumption of more body fluid and *qi*. This condition is often accompanied by some *qi*-deficiency symptoms, such as shortness of breath and lassitude.

3. Since summer also brings rain and therefore dampness, pathogenic summer-heat often invades the body together with pathogenic dampness, clinically marked by some summer-heat symptoms and by some dampness ones as well, such as lassitude in the limbs, stuffy sensation in the chest, nausea, and vomiting.

The Damp Pathogen. Dampness, prevalent in the long summer, is also very common in other seasons. Dampness in excess and causing disease is said to be pathogenic dampness. It possesses the following features:

1. *Yin* in nature, dampness is prone to disturb visceral functions and damage *yang-qi*. As a pathogenic factor, it is substantial, heavy, turbid, and stagnant in nature. Therefore, its invasion most likely promotes disturbance in the visceral functions, retards the ascending, descending, incoming and outgoing functions and stagnates *yang-qi*. These conditions result in the symptoms of stuffiness and distention in the epigastrium and abdomen, nausea, vomiting, diarrhea, etc. Because the spleen is in charge of transporting and transforming fluid, excessive dampness inside the body is liable to disturb the function of spleen-*yang*, thereby resulting in retention of water in the body, which in turn promotes generation of more dampness inside the body.

2. In addition, since dampness is a pathogen that is *yin* in nature, an excess of *yin* may lead to disorder of *yang*. Therefore, the damp pathogen also often impairs the body's *yang-qi*. 2. Heaviness and turbidity characterize dampness. The invasion of dampness in the body often gives rise to such symptoms as heaviness in the head as if it were tightly bound, numbness and heaviness in the joints, as well as turbid (foul) excretions and secretions. For example, the syndrome of arthritis manifested by fixed pain, numbness, and heaviness in the limbs and joints is generally known as damp anthralgia. Such symptoms as excessive secretions in the eyes, dirty complexion, pus-bloody stool, turbid urine, and massive leukorrhea and eczema are characteristic of diseases due to invasion of the damp pathogen.

3. Disease due to dampness is also characterized by viscosity and stagnation. This condition refers to:

    • Damp syndrome marked by stickiness such as slimy and greasy stool and urine and greasy fur of the tongue.

    • A lingering disease difficult to cure, characterized by longer duration of an illness or repeated attacks, as often seen in eczema.

The Dry Pathogen. Dryness, prevalent in autumn, can also be seen in other seasons. Dryness in excess and causing disease is known as pathogenic dryness. It possesses the following features:

1. Pathogenic dryness is liable to impair body fluid. The consumption of body fluid due to invasion by pathogenic dryness promotes a morbid condition due to consumption of *yin* and body fluid. This condition is marked by dryness and cracked skin, dry mouth with cracked lips, dryness of nasal cavity and throat, and dry stool.

2. Since the lungs, as one of the delicate *zang* organs, prefer purity and moistness rather than dryness, pathogenic dryness tends to impair the lungs. Additionally, dry pathogens enter the body through the mouth and nose since they "communicate" with the external atmosphere and the lungs. This condition is marked by such symptoms as dry cough, sticky phlegm difficult to be coughed up, phlegm with blood, and gasping pain in the chest.

The Fire (Heat) Pathogen. Fire-heat, brought about by an excess of *yang*, is often interchangeably called fire or heat. The characteristics of the fire-heat pathogen are summarized as follows.

1. As a pathogenic agent of *yang* nature, the fire pathogen is scorching in nature and its manifestations are high fever, scorching heat, dysphoria, thirst, sweating, red tongue with yellow coating, and a full pulse. Fire tends to flare up; that is to say, the symptoms caused by fire tend to appear in the upper portion of the body. For example, the flaring-up of the heart-fire shows fire symptoms of the heart channel marked by oral ulceration and that of the liver-fire presents such symptoms as conjunctival congestion with painful swelling and mental disturbance due to flaring-up fire pathogen. It is often accompanied by coma and delirium.

2. The fire pathogen is apt to consume *qi* and body fluid. It tends to dispel body fluid and burn and consume *yin*-fluid, clinically manifested by thirst with an inclination for drink and a dry mouth and throat. The outflow of body fluid also results in consumption of *qi*. Moreover, fire-pathogen tends to impair vital *qi* thus leading to general hypofunction and overfatigue.

3. The fire pathogen is liable to stir up wind and disturb blood circulation. Invasion by the fire pathogen often burns the liver channel, exhausts *yin*-fluid and results in malnutrition of the tendons and channels, thus stirring up the liver. This is what is known as the occurrence of wind syndrome from extreme heat. Its clinical manifestations are high fever accompanied by coma and delirium. Furthermore, the fire pathogen may speed up blood flow, burn the channels and collaterals, or even cause

extravasation of blood, thereby bringing about various types of hemorrhage.

4. Pathogenic dryness tends to cause painful swelling on the body surface. Accumulated in a local spot, the fire pathogen is apt to bring about the stagnation of *qi* and blood. Meanwhile, excessive fire damages muscles and blood, thus resulting in large carbuncles and painful swelling on the body surface. These swellings may be localized and one may experience burning pain in the wound or even ulcerations in it.

***Li Qi* (Epidemic Pathogenic Factor).** *Li qi,* the epidemic pathogen is a highly infectious exogenic pathogen, which also bears the names *du qi* (poisonous *qi*) and *yi qi* (extraordinary *qi*). Following are some special features of the epidemic pathogenic factor:

1. It is obviously infectious and epidemic. Epidemic pathogens are spread through the air or by contact and enter the body by way of the mouth and nose. Once infected, one infects other persons susceptible to the infection and the epidemic disease spreads rapidly in the community, thus leading to its onset among large population.

2. The onset of epidemic disease is sudden, its transmission and progress rapid and its morbid conditions severe and fierce.

6.7 INTERNAL IMPAIRMENT BY SEVEN EMOTIONS

According to TCM, the seven emotions refer to joy, anger, melancholy, meditation, grief, fear, and terror. They are emotional responses of the body to environmental stimuli and are normal mental activities. They do not cause disease under normal conditions. However, when sudden, violent, and persistent emotional stimuli exceed the body's ability to adapt and endure, they give rise to dysfunction of the *qi* and blood in the *zang-fu* organs and imbalance between *yin* and *yang* and thus become pathogenic. This condition is known as internal impairment by seven emotions.

Emotions and *Qi* and Blood in the Internal Organs. Emotions are closely related to *qi* and blood in the internal organs. Briefly speaking, emotional activities originate from *qi* and blood in the five *zang* organs, but emotional stress can also impair their *qi* and blood.

On the one hand, the functional activities of the *zang-fu* organs bring about relevant changes in emotions. The chapter "Treatise on Y*in-Yang* Classification of Natural Phenomena" by Su Wen states: "Man has five organs with which to generate five *qi*, from which arise the five emotions, namely, joy, anger, anxiety, melancholy, and fear."

Since the *zang-fu* organs create emotion, they can, on the other hand, promote abnormal emotional activities via dysfunction of *qi* and blood. For instance, anger is exhibited when the liver's control of the normal flow of *qi* is impaired.

On the other hand, emotional stress, acting on the relevant *zang* organ, causes its dysfunction, disorder of *qi*, and irregular flow of blood. Rage impairs the liver, causing adverse and upward flow of *qi* and blood.

Features of Seven Emotions as Pathogenic Factors. The characteristics of seven emotions as pathogenic factors are as follows:

1. They directly affect five *zang* organs and, first of all, heart-*qi*. Unlike the six exogenic pathogenic factors, which invade the body through the mouth, nose, and skin pores, the seven emotions cause disease by directly acting on corresponding internal organs. The heart, as the commanding *zang-fu* organ, houses the mind. Emotional impairment first affects heart-*qi* and then other organs. For example, excessive anxiety may cause retention of heart-*qi* and give rise to accumulation of spleen-*qi*.

2. The seven emotions as pathogens affect the functional activities of *zang-fu* organs. For example, anger injures the liver and rage causes adverse or smooth flow of liver-*qi*. Likewise, joy impairs the heart and excessive joy tends to cause unsteadiness of heart-*qi* and mental derangement, while anxiety impairs the spleen and excessive anxiety leads to accumulation of spleen-*qi* and anorexia. Additionally, fear impairs the kidneys and lungs and excessive fear gives rise to the dispersion of kidney-*qi* and incontinence of urine and stool; melancholy injures the lungs and excessive melancholy leads to the insufficient lung-*qi*, shortness of breath, and weakness of muscles. Finally, terror impairs the heart and excessive terror promotes dysfunction of heart-*qi* causing utter shock of all of the six vital organs.

3. Fluctuations in emotional activities may affect or aggravate some morbid conditions. In the course of a disease, any fluctuation in patients' emotions often aggravate their conditions or even abruptly deteriorates them.

6.8 IMPROPER DIET

Improper diet, such as eating too little, overeating, unsanitary food, and food preference, is often the factor predisposing to disease. Insufficient nourishment intake due to underfeeding promotes lack of the source of *qi* and blood. Furthermore, a prolonged period of under-nourishment results in malnutrition and insufficient *qi* and blood—of course resulting in disease. Additionally, insufficient *qi* and blood gives rise to deficient vital *qi* and lowered body resistance, both of which are easily followed by other disorders.

On the other hand, excessive nourishment due to overeating exceeds the ability of the spleen and stomach to transport and transform it, also causes disease. This condition is marked by symptoms such as indigestion, epigastric distention, belching with fetid odor and nausea, anorexia, vomiting, diarrhea. The chapter "On Stagnation-Syndrome of *Qi* and Blood" by Su Wen states: "Overeating tends to impair the gastrointestinal organs." Similarly, the intake of unsanitary food also causes many different gastrointestinal diseases—or parasitic ones—manifested in abdominal pain, vomiting, and diarrhea.

Additionally, the intake of stale food or food containing poison usually promotes symptoms such as severe abdominal pain, vomiting, and diarrhea and even coma or death in severe cases.

Finally, preference for super-heated or super-cooled food or habitual preference for one of the five flavors may result in imbalance between *yin* and *yang* or disorders due to malnutrition.

6.9 IMBALANCE BETWEEN WORK AND REST

Imbalance between work and rest, may also turn out to be a pathogenic factor. Again, overwork can be classified into three types:
- Undue physical exertion
- Undue mental exertion
- Intemperance in sexual life

Undue physical exertion refers to constant overwork that can wear you down and impair and exhaust *qi*. Undue mental work refers to excessive meditation or anxiety which can impair the heart and spleen. Too much mental work will consume heart-blood and impair spleen-*qi*, thereby producing such symptoms as palpitation due to denutrition of the heart, insomnia, amnesia, anorexia, and abdominal distention. Finally, intemperance in sexual life refers to excessive sexual activity, which results in consumption of kidney-essence accompanied by lassitude in the loins and knees, vertigo, tinnitus, listlessness, and sexual hypofunction such as spermatorrhea,prospermia,and impotence.

6.10 TRAUMATIC INJURY

Included in this section are gunshot injuries, incised wounds, contusions, sprains, scalds and burns, cold injury, and injury inflicted by animal stings or bites.

Such traumatic injuries as gunshot injuries, incised wounds, contusions, sprains and others may lead to blood stasis and painful swelling on the skin and muscles, bleeding or laceration of muscles and tendons, fractures, and dislocations. In serious cases, internal organs may be affected resulting in *yang* depletion and prostration syndrome may occur as a result of massive hemorrhage.

Burns and scalds are usually caused by high temperature objects, boiling water, scorching oil or fire. Slight burns and scalds only injure the skin and manifest as redness, swelling, fever or pain in the affected area while severe ones are complicated by such symptoms as dysphoria, fever, thirst or oliguria or even death due to severe pain in the wound, internal invasion by fire-toxin, and evaporation of body fluids.

Cold injury refers to general or local traumatic wound due to attack of low temperatures. Cold injury results from failure of *yang-qi* to warm the body and to promote blood circulation due to its impairment and consumption by cold pathogens. Symptomatically, cold injuries are accompanied by gradual lowering of the body temperature, pale face, bluish purple lips, tongue and finger nails, shallow breathing slow and faint pulse. Its clinical manifestations are local pale skin and cold numbness, followed by swelling and itching pain and scorching heat or blisters of various size.

Insect or animal stings and bites include bites by poisonous snakes, wild beasts, rabid dogs or stings by scorpions and bees. In, mild cases, local injury occurs, accompanied by painful swelling and bleeding. In severe cases, however, some of the internal organs may be involved or even death ensues as a result of massive hemorrhage.

6.11 PHLEGM RETENTION

Phlegm retention is a pathological product resulting from disturbance in water metabolism. It is also referred to as a pathogenic factor because after its formation it may act directly or indirectly upon certain parts of the body, producing some new pathological changes in *zang-fu* organs and tissues manifested by various symptoms and signs. The phlegm-retention refers not only to the retention of phlegm but to water retention as well. Phlegm retention is further subdivided into tangible and formless. Tangible fluid is a kind of mucoid substance visible, palpable, or vocal. Formless is an invisible fluid stagnating in *zang-fu* and channel tissues. It presents clinical manifestations, which can be determined and cured with an expectorant.

Formation of Phlegm Retention. Phlegm retention is formed by an accumulation of water-dampness due to dysfunction of the lungs, spleen, kidneys, and tri-*jiao* resulting from invasion by the six exogenic pathogenic factors. These organs and tri-*jiao* are closely related to circulation, distribution and the excretion of water and fluid. As an example, the spleen governs the transportation and transformation of water and fluid in the body. The lungs perform dispersing, purifying and descending functions, regulate water passages and promote diffusion of body fluid. The kindeys dominate water metabolism, in which clean fluid is retained and turbid fluid flows down into the urinary bladder as excretion. The coordination among functions of the spleen,lungs and kidneys and unobstructed water passages in the region of tri-*jiao* leads to distribution of nutrients to all parts of the body and simultaneous functioning of the five main channels. When dysfunction of the spleen, lungs, kidneys and tri-*jiao* occurs, the body fluid stagnates and accumulates to form phlegm.

Pathogenic Characteristics of Phlegm Retention. When phlegm is formed, it flows together with *qi* to all parts of the body. Its pathogenic characteristics are summarized as follows:

1. It obstructs the circulation of *qi* and blood in the channels and vessels. The retention of phlegm in the channels may block the circulation of *qi* and blood, thus causing numbness of limbs. If phlegm accumulates in the heart, it obstructs circulation of heart-blood which results in a choking sensation in the chest and palpitations.

2. It prevents the *qi* from ascending or descending by flowing into the *zang-fu* organs. For example, stomach-phlegm may cause the failure of stomach-*qi* to descend and manifests symptoms such as serious vomiting or fullness in the stomach.

3. It affects water metabolism. Phlegm is formed by a disturbance in water metabolism. Once stagnated, it can interfere with the ascending and descending functions of *qi*. Since *qi* promotes the circulation of water, stagnation of *qi* leads to retention of water in the body, which in turn, further aggravates disturbance in water metabolism.

4. It tends to disturb mental activities. Stagnation of phlegm in the heart may block the heart orifice and bring about impairment of mental activities, marked by such symptoms as coma and dementia. What is more, manic-depressive psychosis may also occur as a result of mental disturbance due to phlegm-fire.

6.12 BLOOD STASIS

Blood stasis is a pathological product resulting from abnormal circulation and stagnation of blood. It refers to the blood accumulated within the body and the blood stagnated in channels, vessels, and *zang-fu* organs due to impeded blood circulation. Its formation may further influence the circulation of *qi* and blood, thereby bringing about dysfunction of *zang-fu* tissues accompanied by a variety of symptoms. Consequently, it is also considered as a pathogenic factor.

Formation of Blood Stasis. The factors contributing to blood stasis are numerous and varied, but it is due chiefly to stagnation of *qi*, deficient *qi*, blood-cold, and blood-heat. It can be formed either by accumulation of stagnant blood in certain spots due to impeded blood circulation or by inability of blood to be dispersed or eliminated due to internal bleeding as a result of traumatic injury. The main contributing factors are listed as follows:

1. Stagnation of *qi* may result from the impairment of emotions, accumulation of liver-*qi*, or disturbance in functional activities of *qi*.

2. Deficient *qi*. Deficient *qi* leads to slow transportation and sluggish blood flow thereby resulting in blood stasis.

3. Blood-cold refers to pathogenic cold or excessive *yin* cold due to deficient *yang* and stagnation of blood.

4. Blood-heat refers to the invasion of the blood system by heat that exhausts *yin* and stagnates the blood. Blood-heat also refers to an accumulation of blood in the *zang-fu* organs and tissues without timely dispersion due to injury of superficial venules.

5. Blood stasis can also form due to bleeding from traumatic injury. Contusions, sprains, squeezing, and pressing can externally injure muscles and internally impair *zang-fu* organs.

6. Improper diet can also lead to blood stasis. Improper diet may impair the collateral branches of the large channels in the intestines and stomach.

Pathological Characteristics of Blood Stasis. When blood stasis is formed, systemic or local circulation is hindered, thereby producing various syndromes. Its main pathological characteristics can be summed up as follows:

1. The pain blood stasis causes may be described as a stabbing pain that is confined to a fixed area. It is usually milder during the day than in the night.

2. A lump on the body surface may appear that is a bluish-purple color, limited to a fixed location and tender on pressure.

3. Bleeding can occur with blood that is dark purplish in color; it can be mixed with clots.

4. Cyanosis is usually seen on the face, mouth and lips and fingernails. It assumes the form of purplish spots on the skin or the tongue accompanied by a thready, hesitant and taut pulse.

6.13 VITAL *QI*

Vital *qi*, also known as genuine *qi*, refers to the body's functional activities and disease-resistant and rehabilitating capabilities. Such activities include its adaptation to the natural environment, defense against exogenic pathogens, self-repair of injuries, as well as readjustment to functional disturbances.

Insufficient Vital *Qi* as the Intrinsic Factor in the Cause of Disease. A disease is the outcome of a struggle between pathogenic factors and vital *qi*. Insufficient vital *qi* is the intrinsic factor in the onset of a disease. When vital *qi* is sufficient, it is difficult for pathogens to invade the body, thus, disease cannot occur. However, when vital *qi* is insufficient to resist the invasion of pathogens, they manage to enter the body and cause disease.

Pathogens are said to be the predominant factor in the cause of disease. A disease may occur if there are too many pathogens for vital *qi* to overcome because its resistance is rather limited. For example, epidemic pathogenic factors, traumatic injury, and others often play a leading role in the cause of disease independent of the condition of vital *qi*.

The struggle between vital *qi* and pathogens not only causes disease, but it influences its development and termination. When pathogens invade the body, vital *qi* immediately rushes to the site of invasion to fight them off. If vital *qi* is powerful enough to guard against invasion, it is very hard for pathogens to get into the body. That is why not all persons exposed to various kinds of pathogens in nature contract disease. This is said to be an outcome of the victory of vital *qi* over pathogens.

When a disease occurs, it manifests itself by different syndromes, depending on the disease-resisting power of the vital *qi* within the body, the virulence of the invading pathogens, the severity of the disease, and the part of the body it is affecting. For instance, an excess syndrome occurs when vital *qi* is powerful enough to destroy pathogens in desperate struggle against them. A deficiency syndrome occurs when vital *qi* is insufficient or too weak to resist pathogens. In general, a slight invasion by pathogens leads to mild disorders while serious invasion by pathogens leads to severe ones.

Moreover, diseases vary with the locations or parts affected. For example, attack of the skin by pathogens generally presents exterior syndromes whereas invasion of the *zang-fu* organs produces interior ones. Exterior invasion by pathogens leads to mild and superficial disorders while interior invasion, to deep and serious ones.

6.14 ENVIRONMENT AS A FACTOR IN THE CAUSE OF DISEASE

Disease occurrence is closely related to one's internal and external environment. External environment refers mainly to your living and working surroundings, including climactic variations, geographical features, and environmental sanitation. Our human condition readily adapts to the external environment in order to survive. Abnormal changes in natural and working surroundings predispose humans to disease.

Internal environment mainly refers to the vital *qi* of the body. The strength of vital *qi* is closely linked with the body's constitutional and mental state. For instance, a strong and vigorous constitution is a manifestation of sufficient vital *qi*, while a weak or feeble constitution is a manifestation of deficient vital *qi*. A strong constitution relies on ones diet, nutrition, and physical exercise.

Joyful emotions and mental happiness also bring about a balance between *qi*, blood, the *zang-fu* organs, and vital *qi*. Sad emotions and mental depression can lead to an imbalance between *yin* and *yang* and *qi* and blood, dysfunction of *zang-fu* organs, and weakened vital *qi*. Therefore, a strong resistance to disease usually accompanies a sturdy constitution and happy emotions.

CHAPTER 7

Pathogenesis

7.1 PATHOGENESIS

Pathogenesis is the mechanism of occurrence, development and change of a disease. Pathogenesis is closely related to the strength of the body's vital *qi* and nature of the invading pathogenic factors. For example, the invasion of *yang* pathogens tends to consume the body's *yin*-fluid while the invasion of *yin* pathogens impairs the body's *yang-qi*. This disturbs the relative balance between *yin* and *yang*. As a result of this imbalance the *zang-fu* organs and channels and collaterals can become dysfunctional, as well as the *qi* and blood. This in turn can bring about a variety of general or local pathological changes that manifest in ever changing clinical symptoms. Therefore, the general pathogenesis of a disease is inseparable from the wax or wane of vital *qi* and pathogens, the imbalance between *yin* and *yang*, the disorder of *qi* and blood and the dysfunction of *zang-fu* organs and channels and collaterals.

7.2 WAX OR WANE OF VITAL *QI* AND PATHOGENS

The wax or wane of vital *qi* and pathogens refers to the struggle between vital *qi* and invading pathogens in the onset of a disease. The constant struggle between them is not only prevalent during the cause of disease but during the recovery period as well. The wax and wane of pathogens and vital *qi* also determines the nature of pathological changes such as the excess syndrome or deficiency syndrome.

Excess Syndrome. Su Wen states, "An excess syndrome results when the invading pathogens are exuberant." That is to say that although the invading pathogens are excessive, the body's defensive *qi* does not decline. As a result, a fierce struggle between them creates a series of pathological reactions of excess known as excess syndrome. This syndrome is often observed in the early or middle stages of an exogenic disease due to stagnation of phlegm, food, blood or water in the body. Its clinical manifestations are high fever, mania, high voice and strong breath, abdominal pain and tenderness, and constipation. Additionally there may be some morbid conditions marked by excessive accumulation of phlegm and fluid-retention, indigestion of food, reverse flow of water within the body and stagnant blood.

Deficiency Syndrome. Su Wen also comments on deficiency syndrome stating, "Exhaustion of vital essence promotes deficiency syndrome." Deficiency syndrome refers to deficient vital *qi*—a pathological reaction with deficient vital *qi* as the principal aspect of the contradiction. That is to say, when vital *qi* is exhausted, *yin* and *yang*, *qi* and blood are all insufficient. The *zang-fu* organs and channels and collaterals fail to function properly and the body resistance is lowered while the pathogens are no longer excessive or are declining. During this time a struggle between vital *qi* and invading pathogens is ongoing. This struggle is followed by a series of pathological reactions of deficiency, known as deficiency syndrome, and is seen primarily in debilitated patients, in the later stage of a disease, and in many chronic cases. Deficiency syndrome displays the following symptoms.

- Lassitude and a thin and pallid complexion
- Palpitations
- Shortness of breath
- Spontaneous perspiration
- Night sweats

A Combination of Deficiency and Excess Syndromes. The wax or wane of vital *qi* and pathogens can bring about excess syndrome or deficiency syndrome, but it can also bring about pathological changes a mixture of the two. A combination of excess and deficiency syndromes is comprised of mainly two kinds of pathological changes:
- Deficiency syndromes complicated with excess syndromes.
- Excess syndromes complicated with deficiency syndromes.

Deficiency syndromes complicated with excess syndromes often result from an inability to fight off pathogens due to insufficient vital *qi* or due to stagnation of such pathological products as phlegm, food, blood, and water within the body. Excess syndromes complicated with deficiency syndromes are caused by impairment of vital *qi* due to long term invasion by pathogens. A combination of excess and deficiency syndromes is an inevitable tendency in the development of some diseases.

Genuine or Pseudo-Excess or Deficiency Syndrome. The genuine or pseudo-excess or deficiency syndrome falls under two types of pathological changes:
- Genuine excess with pseudo-deficiency syndrome.
- Genuine deficiency with pseudo-excess syndrome.

The appearance of genuine excess with pseudo-deficiency symptom, also known as deficiency in extreme excess, is caused by an obstruction of the channels and collaterals, which causes a failure to transport *qi* and blood outward due to accumulation of heat in the intestine and stomach. It is accompanied by a fecal impaction due to heat with watery discharge.

Genuine deficiency with pseudo-excess syndrome, also known as symptoms of excess in extreme deficiency, usually results from the dysfunction of the *zang-fu* organs and their failure to transport and transform nutrients. It is usually accompanied by abdominal distention due to dysfunction of the spleen.

Recovery from Disease as a Result of Victory of Vital *Qi* over Pathogens. After the onset of a disease, its recovery or development depends on the outcome of the struggle between vital *qi* and pathogens. The victory of vital *qi* over pathogens tends toward improvement or even complete recovery from the disease. This is because the vital *qi* is sufficient and resistance against the pathogens is rather strong, resulting in complete recovery. For example, febrile disease is caused by exogenic pathogens. If vital *qi* is sufficient and exerts powerful resistance against those pathogens that invade the body through skin pores or via the mouth or nose, it will:

- Slow down further development of a disease

- Confine the lesions to superficial muscles or to channels and collaterals

- Expel the pathogens by means of its action on them

Once superficial syndrome is relieved, harmony between nutritive and defensive *qi* is reestablished and the disease ends in a complete cure.

Development of Disease as a Result of Victory of Pathogens over Vital *Qi*. As mentioned earlier, recovery due to the victory of vital *qi* over pathogens is a common termination of a number of disorders, but if the pathogens are sufficient and vital *qi* deficient, this will not be the case. When vital *qi* is deficient and pathogens are excessive and the body's resistance against such pathogens weakens, vital *qi* has difficulty checking their pathogenic action; thus, pathological lesions inflicted on the body get more serious. If vital *qi* is exhausted, *qi* and blood, *zang-fu* organs and channels and collaterals all fail to function properly, resulting in dissociation of *yin* and *yang* and death.

7.3 IMBALANCE BETWEEN *YIN* AND *YANG*

Imbalance between *yin* and *yang* refers to the morbid state resulting from the breakdown in the equilibrium of *yin-yang* in the body. In the course of the occurrence and development of a disease, the body loses its relative balance and harmony between *yin* and *yang* due to the action of various invading pathogens. In turn this leads to such morbid conditions as relative excessiveness or deficient *yin* and *yang*, mutual impairment, an abnormally strong pulse, and exhaustion of *yin* and *yang*.

An imbalance of *yin* and *yang* can be regarded as a summary of any dysfunction in these interrelations: The *zang-fu* organs, channels and collaterals, *qi* and blood, nutritive and defensive *qi*, the functions of ascending or descending and the intake or output of *qi*. Additionally, disease is a life process in which pathogens act on the body to bring about imbalance between *yin* and *yang*—the basic pathogenesis and general principle of pathology in TCM.

Imbalance between *yin* and *yang* is primarily manifested by such pathological changes as cold or heat, excess or deficiency syndrome and genuine, pseudo-excess, or pseudo-deficiency syndromes. "Cold or heat syndrome determined by imbalance between *yin* and *yang*."

Relative Excessiveness of *Yin* or *Yang*. Relative excessiveness of *yin* or *yang* may lead to an excess syndrome resulting from exuberant invading pathogens. Depending on the kind of pathogens that invade the body, specific syndromes may occur. For example, the invasion of *yang* pathogens results in the relative excessiveness of *yang* and thus leads to a heat syndrome of excess type; excessiveness of *yin* pathogens gives rise to the relative excessiveness of *yin* and leads to an interior cold syndrome of excess type. Su Wen states: "An excess of *yang* promotes heat syndrome and that of *yin*, cold syndrome."

Yin and *yang* are mutually "restrainable" in that growth of *yang* leads to the consumption of *yin*, while that of *yin* to the consumption of *yang*. Su Wen says, "An excess of *yang* leads to disorder of *yin* and that of *yin*, to disorder of *yang*," and certainly points out the inevitable trend of the relative excessiveness of *yin* or *yang*.

Heat Syndrome Due to an Excess of *Yang*. The main reason for excessive *yang* is that the body is affected by warm-heat *yang* pathogens or by *yin* pathogens with heat transformed from excess *yang*. An excess of *yang* can also result from interior impairment by emotional stress (disorders of the five emotions) or from the stagnation of *qi* and blood— all of which are transformed into heat pathogens. Other causes of heat syndrome of the excess type include a preponderance of *yang-qi* and the hyperfunction and production of excessive heat. An excess of *yang* is characterized by heat, movement, and dryness and is inevitably accompanied by such heat syndromes as high fever, flushed face, and congested eyes.

Because *yin* and *yang* are mutually opposite, an excess of *yang* leads inevitably to consumption of *yin*. When pathogens associated with *yang* cause an excess of *yang*, *yin* is relatively inadequate and a heat syndrome of excess type occurs. When excessive *yang* consumes the body's *yin*-fluid, *yin* is absolutely inadequate. The result of this inadequacy is excessive heat syndrome complicated by *yin* deficiency or by developing into a *yin* deficiency syndrome.

Cold Syndrome Due to an Excess of *Yin*. "A cold syndrome brought about by an excess of *yin*" displays interior cold syndrome of the excess type due to excessiveness of *yin* in the body. An excess of *yin* is primarily caused by *yin* pathogenic cold and dampness, profuse intake of cold or raw food, or retention of cold and fluid in the middle-*jiao* due to stagnant cold. Hence, inhibition of *yang-qi* due to relative excessive-ness of *yin* may produce some pathological metabolic products such as stagnant phlegm and accumulated blood, thereby giving rise to a cold syndrome of the excess type. An excess of *yin* marked by cold, inertia, and dampness is almost always followed by such cold symptoms as chilliness, cold limbs, and pale tongue.

Much like the effects of excess *yang* on *yin*, an excess of *yin* is bound to consume *yang-qi*. Theoretically, relative inadequacy of *yang* is a cold syndrome of excess type; absolute inadequacy of *yang* is an excessive cold syndrome complicated by *yang* deficiency. Because *yang-qi* is liable to move and easy to be dispersed out, the excessiveness of *yin* is simultane-ously accompanied by *yang* inadequacy in varying degrees. Clinically, it is very hard to make a clear distinction between the relative inadequacy and absolute inadequacy of *yang*, or to distinguish pure cold syndrome of excess type from that complicated by *yang* deficiency syndrome.

Relative Deficient *Yin* or *Yang*. Relative deficient *yin* or *yang* leads to deficiency syndrome brought about by exhaustion of vital essence. Exhaustion of vital essence includes deficient some basic substances such as essences of life, *qi*, blood, and the fluids of the body, as well as physiological hypofunction of the essences, *zang-fu* organs, channels, and collaterals. In normal circumstances, mutual restraint, interdependence, mutual growth-decline, and mutual transformation between *yin* and *yang* exist and thus maintain relative balance between *yin* and *yang*. The relationships between *yin* and *yang* explain the body organs and structures such as essence of life, *qi*, blood, body fluid, *zang-fu* organs and channels and collaterals and their physiological functions. If for one reason or another, a reduction of *yin* or *yang*—or the hypo-function of either—exists, one aspect does not restrain the other. This condition results in relative excessiveness of either *yin* or *yang* and morbid conditions marked by a cold syndrome due to *yang* deficiency (cold of insufficiency type) or by a heat syndrome due to *yin* deficiency (heat of insufficiency type).

Cold Syndrome Due to *Yang* Deficiency. Cold syndrome due to *yang* deficiency is a generalization of the pathogenesis of insufficient body's *yang-qi* and production of endogenic cold of deficiency type. The inadequacy of *yang-qi* is usually caused by poor natural endowments, improper diet after birth, internal injury due to over-fatigue, or consumption of *yang-qi* due to chronic illness. If *yang-qi* is inadequate, it cannot restrain *yin* and thus gives rise to relative excessiveness of *yin* and production of endogenic cold of deficiency type. Moreover, if *yang-qi* is deficient, decline of its warming function results in:

- Dysfunction of *zang-fu* organs, channels, and collaterals
- Slow flow of blood and body fluid
- Excess endogenic *yin* cold due to retention of water and fluid
- Deficiency symptoms such as huddling up of the body with preference for inertia or diarrhea with undigested food in the stool
- Cold symptoms such as pale complexion, aversion to cold, cold limbs, pale tongue, and slow pulse

Heat Syndrome Due to *Yin* Deficiency. Heat syndrome due to *yin* deficiency is a generalization of the pathogenesis of inadequacy of the body's *yin*-fluid (including essence of life, blood, and body fluid) and production of endogenic heat of deficiency type. The inadequacy of the body's *yin*-fluid results mostly from impairment of *yin* by *yang*-heat pathogens, by fire transformed from five emotions in excess or by exhaustion of *yin*-fluid due to chronic illness. If *yin* fluid is insufficient, it cannot restrain *yang*, thus resulting in the relative excessiveness of *yang*, debilitating hyperactivity and production of endogenic heat-fire of the deficiency type. This morbid condition due to *yin* deficiency clinically manifests as dysphoria with feverish sensation in the chest palms and soles, hectic fever and tidal fever, night sweats, dry throat and mouth, reddened tongue with little or no fur, and thready and rapid pulse.

Mutual Impairment of *Yin* and *Yang*. Mutual impairment refers to the pathogenesis in which, when either *yin* or *yang* is impaired, its pathological changes affect its opposite aspect, thus leading to deficient *yin* and *yang*.

Yin deficiency followed by *yang* deficiency is known as deficient *yin* affecting *yang*. Conversely, *yang* deficiency followed by *yin* deficiency is named deficient *yang* affecting *yin*. Morbid conditions due to *yang* deficiency affecting *yin* or vice versa occur only because of the imbalance between kidney *yin* and *yang*. This imbalance is due to the deficient *yin* or *yang* of the other *zang* organs or of the kidneys themselves, for the kidneys are the foundation of *yin*-fluid and *yang-qi* of the whole body.

Deficient *Yin* Affecting *Yang*. Deficient *yin* affecting *yang* denotes the pathogenesis of deficient *yin* and *yang* with *yin* deficiency as the primary deficiency. *Yang* cannot be generated without *yin*, so consumption of *yin*-essence leads to insufficient *yang-qi* or loss of the carrier upon which it depends, thereby causing the dispersion of *yang-qi*. This condition is often seen in the case of hyperactivity of liver-*yang*. Its pathogenesis is chiefly characterized by hyperactivity of *yang* due to *yin* deficiency caused by failure of water to nourish wood, but its further development may again consume kidney-*yin* with kidney-*yang* involved. As a result, a *yang* deficiency syndrome marked by aversion to cold, cold limbs, deep and weak pulse may occur and develop into the syndrome of deficient *yin* and *yang*, caused by deficient *yin* affecting *yang*.

Deficient *Yang* Affecting *Yin*. Deficient *yang* affecting *yin* represents the pathogenesis of deficient *yin* and *yang*, although *yin* deficiency is primary. Impairment of *yang-qi* leads to inadequate production of *yin*-essence. This condition is often seen in the case of edema. Its pathogenesis is mainly marked by deficient *yang-qi*, leading to dysfunction in *qi* transportation, disturbance in water metabolism, and stagnation of body fluid. These conditions result in the production of endogenic water and dampness that flow over the skin and muscles, and its development may lead to ever-increasing consumption of *yin* due to an absence of the generation of *yang*. As a result, *yin* deficiency syndrome—marked by emaciation and irritability with the sensation of flaming up of fire— often occurs and may further develop into deficient *yin* and *yang* brought about by deficient *yang* involving *yin*.

Geju (Opposition and Exclusion) of *Yin* and *Yang*. *Geju* of *yin* and *yang* denotes that *yin* and *yang* oppose and exclude each other, causing the pathogenesis of genuine or pseudo-cold or pseudo-heat syndrome, which is a comparatively specific imbalance between yin and yang. When extremely excessive, *yin* or *yang* stagnates inside the body, expels the opposite aspect from it, and makes *yin* and *yang* unable to hold each other together. This condition results in a cold syndrome with pseudo-heat symptoms or a heat syndrome with pseudo-cold symptoms. To sum up, the pathogenesis of opposition and exclusion of yin and yang comprises two aspects:

1. *Yang* kept externally by *yin*-excess in the interior.
2. *Yin* kept externally by *yang*-excess in the interior.

Yang Kept Externally by Yin-Excess in the Interior. The expression "*yang* kept externally by *yin*-excess in the interior" or simply "*yang* kept externally" is a generalization of the pathogenesis of a cold syndrome with pseudo-heat symptoms. Stagnation of excessive *yin*-cold inside the body compels *yang-qi* to flow externally and makes *yin* and *yang* unable to communicate by keeping each other apart. This condition thereby produces a cold syndrome with pseudo-heat symptoms. Of course, excessive *yin*-cold inside the body is the essence of disease. Yet because *yang* is kept externally, such pseudo-heat symptoms as flushed face, dysphoria with smothery sensation, thirst, and large pulse, are likely to occur.

Yin Kept Externally by Yang-Excess in the Interior. The expression "*yin* kept externally by *yang*-excess in the interior" or simply "*yin* kept externally" is a generalization of the pathogenesis of a heat syndrome with pseudo-cold symptoms. Blocked inside the body, extreme *yang*-heat cannot be transported externally to the limbs; *yin* is kept externally so that *yin* and *yang* cannot communicate with each other, thereby producing a heat syndrome with pseudo-cold symptoms. Here, excessive *yang*-heat inside the body is the essence of disease. Yet because *yin* is kept externally, there may appear such pseudo-cold symptoms as cold limbs and deep and hidden pulse.

Finally, when *yin* and *yang* are dissociated from each other, vital essence and *qi* are exhausted and, as a result, all life activities cease to go on and death ensues.

Yin Depletion. *Yin* depletion is a morbid state in which sudden massive consumption or loss of *yin*-fluid leads to severe overall function failure. Generally speaking, *yin* depletion is caused by an excess of pathogenic heat or its long stagnation leading to decocting and burning of much body fluid or by massive loss of *yin*-fluid resulting from profuse sweating, severe vomiting, or massive bleeding. *Yin* depletion is often accompanied by some critical symptoms such as dyspnea, thirst, dysphoria, and profuse sweating with warm hands and feet.

Yang Depletion. *Yang* depletion is a morbid state in which sudden exhaustion of *yang-qi* leads to an abrupt and severe overall functional failure. Generally, *yang* depletion is caused by sudden exhaustion of *yang-qi* due to an excess of pathogens that vital *qi* is unable to fight off. It may also result from:

- Deficient *yang*
- Over-fatigue

- Profuse sweat and excretion of *yang* together with sweat.
- *Yang* exhaustion as a result of chronic consumptive diseases.
- External floating of *yang* in deficiency condition. This morbid state is usually manifested by some critical symptoms, such as profuse sweat, cold limbs, and weak indistinct pulse.

7.4 *QI* AND BLOOD

Derangement of *qi* and blood refers to a morbid condition due to insufficient *qi* and blood, abnormality of their respective physiological functions, and dysfunction of their interdependence and interaction. On one hand, *qi* and blood are the material basis for the physiological activities that the *zang-fu* organs, channels and collaterals perform. Therefore, the derangement of *qi* and blood inevitably affects the body's various physiological functions and results in a disease. On the other hand, *qi* and blood are the products of the functional activities of *zang-fu* organs and, therefore, any pathological change they undergo certainly influences *qi* and blood, thus giving rise to pathological changes of *qi* and blood.

Deficient *Qi.* Deficient *qi* is a morbid state due to whole body's consumption of *qi* and its resulting dysfunction, hypofunction of the *zang-fu* organs, and lowered resistance against diseases. The main reason for this condition is inadequate generation and excessive consumption of *qi*. The former results from congenital defect, lack of proper care after birth, or dysfunction of the lungs, spleen, and kidneys; the latter results from internal injury due to over-fatigue or severe protracted illness. Deficient *qi*, leading to hypofunction of various organs, manifests in listlessness, lassitude, spontaneous sweating and susceptibility to cold. Since *qi* bears a close relationship with blood and body fluid, deficient *qi* is bound to affect the generation, transportation, and distribution of blood and body fluid, thereby also giving rise to many pathological changes of blood and body fluid. For instance, deficient *qi* results in:

- An inability to transport blood or diffuse body fluid, thus leading to their stagnation.
- An inability to control blood and body fluid, thereby incurring their loss.
- An inability to generate blood and body fluid.

Disorder of *Qi.*

1. Generally speaking, disorder of *qi* includes the following five pathological changes: Stagnation of *qi* (its impeded circulation).

2. Reversed flow of *qi* (its excessive upward flow and inadequate downward flow).

3. Collapse of *qi* (its inadequate upward flow and excessive downward flow of *qi*).

4. Blockage of *qi* (obstruction of its external flow).

5. Exhaustion of *qi* (its external depletion instead of its retention inside the body).

Ascending-descending and incoming-outgoing movements are the basic motions of *qi*. It is upon these motions that the functional activities of the *zang-fu* organs, channels, and collaterals—and their interrelations—rely for their relative balance. A disturbance in ascending-descending and incoming-outgoing flow of *qi* disturbs their functional coordination and balance and thus promotes the morbid conditions described above.

Stagnation of *Qi*. *Qi* in motion enables blood and body fluid to circulate normally. Stagnation of *qi* is due chiefly to emotional depression or stagnation of products such as phlegm, food, blood, and water—and any of these products, in turn, can cause the production of the other products and the stagnation of *qi*. This condition hinders the flow of *qi*, causes general or local disorders of its functional activities and subsequently results in dysfunction of some *zang-fu* organs, channels and collaterals. For example, localized stagnation of *qi* in a certain spot promotes abdominal distention and pain.

Reversed Flow of *Qi*. Reversed flow of *qi* indicates a morbid condition in which the upward and downward flow of *qi* is disturbed, marked by an upward adverse flow of *qi* of the *zang-fu* organs. This condition is primarily caused by emotional upset, improper cold or warm factors, or stagnation of phlegm and is most frequently found in the lungs, stomach, and liver. As examples:

- Adverse rising of lung-*qi* due to impairment of the lung's purifying and descending function manifests as cough with dyspnea.

- Adverse rising of stomach-*qi* due to its failure in descending results in nausea, vomiting, belching and hiccups.

- The upward invasion of hyperactive liver-*qi* due to its excessive flow manifests as headache, fullness of the head, flushed face, congested eyes, and irritability. (The liver, an energetic *zang-fu* organ, maintains the potency of the flow of *qi* and storage of blood; therefore, upward invasion of the hyperactive liver-*qi* leads to hemoptysis due to the reversed flow of *qi* or even to syncope due to disturbance of *qi* in the brain.) Generally, the reversed flow of *qi* belongs to an excess syndrome, but it is occasionally found in a deficiency syndrome. Impairment of purifying and descending function due to deficiency syndrome of the lungs or failure of the kidneys to adequately receive *qi* leads to the upward flow of *qi*, as often seen in asthma of insufficiency type.

Collapse of *Qi*. Collapse of *qi* is a morbid condition mainly characterized by non-vigorous ascending and descending of *qi*.

Note that the *zang-fu* organs depend on coordination of *qi*'s ascending-descending and incoming-outgoing movements for their fixed positions in the body. Because the spleen, as the source of growth and development of *qi* and blood, performs the function of sending up essential nutrients, its insufficiency is more likely to cause *qi* collapse. This condition usually manifests as some symptoms of the deficiency type, such as abdominal distention with tenesmus, frequent urge to defecate, shortness of breath, listlessness, weak voice, and weak pulse.

Blockage of *Qi*. Blockage of *qi* refers to a morbid state in which the flow of *qi* is suddenly obstructed either by turbid pathogens or by excessive stagnation of *qi*. This condition manifests as syncope, heat in exogenic febrile diseases, and sudden mental disorder.

Exhaustion of *Qi*. Exhaustion of *qi* refers to a morbid state characterized by sudden functional failure of *qi* resulting from the exhaustion of *qi*. External exhaustion of *qi* means that we use too much of our external *qi* and, thus, internal *qi* "leaks" to the outside to replenish what is lost. This condition results from:

- Failure of vital *qi* to ward off pathogens.
- Prolonged weakening of vital *qi*.
- Exhaustion of *qi* caused by massive bleeding or profuse sweat.

Since *qi* is the most fundamental substance to maintain vital functions, the loss of a large amount of *qi* gives rise to sudden failure of visceral function. Exhaustion of *qi* is the leading pathogenesis of various prostration syndromes.

Deficient Blood. Deficient blood refers to a morbid condition due to insufficient blood and hypofunction of its nourishment. This condition is attributable chiefly to an inability to generate blood or the excessive consumption of blood.

Inability to generate blood results from:
- Weakness of the spleen and stomach
- Malnutrition

Excessive consumption results from:
* Massive hemorrhage
* Slow and unconscious consumption of nutritive *qi* and blood due to chronic illness

Since the *zang-fu* organs and tissues, channels, and collaterals depend on blood for their nourishment, deficient blood may lead to weak syndromes of deficiency type, such as general or localized malnutrition and gradual decline of functional activities. Its clinical symptoms are: pale complexion, pale lips, dizziness, palpitation, lassitude, listlessness, emaciation, numbness of the extremities, impeded stretch and contraction of the joints, dryness and uncomfortable feeling of the eyes, and vertigo.

Blood Stasis. Blood stasis refers to a morbid condition caused by obstructed or sluggish blood flow. It is due chiefly to stagnation of *qi*, deficient *qi*, blood-cold, blood-heat, and retention of phlegm in the interior. Specifically:
* Stagnation of *qi* leads to impeded blood circulation.
* Deficient *qi* leads to its sluggish circulation.
* Invasion of blood by cold pathogens leads to coagulation due to blood-cold.
* Invasion of blood by heat pathogens leads to decoction and sticky stagnation.
* Retention of phlegm in the channels and collaterals leads to the obstruction of blood circulation.

Any one of the above five cases is enough to cause blood stasis and even result in stagnant blood. Ironically, since stagnant blood is the pathological product of blood stasis, it may be obstructed in channels and collaterals after its formation, thus serving as yet another cause of blood stasis.

The pathological changes that blood stasis causes are basically similar to those of stagnant blood. Additionally, blood stasis may in turn aggravate the obstruction of *qi*'s functional activities, thereby forming a vicious cycle in which stagnation of *qi* leads to blood stasis and vice versa. Consequently, stagnation of *qi* and blood stasis are often simultaneously seen in the course of a disease.

Blood-Heat. Blood-heat is a morbid state due to heat in the blood system and speeding up of blood flow. It is caused by attack of blood by heat pathogens and by fire pathogen transformed by emotional disorders due to mental depression.

Blood-heat is clinically characterized not only by heat symptoms, but by consumption of blood, bleeding, and impairment of *yin* as well. These symptoms occurs for two reasons:

1. Heat in the blood system and the resulting forced flow of blood may speed up the flow of blood and burn channels and vessels, resulting in various kinds of bleeding.

2. Invasion of blood by heat pathogens decocts blood and body fluid.

***Qi* Stagnation and Blood Stasis.** The morbid condition that is the simultaneous occurrence of stagnation of *qi* and blood stasis falls into one of three types:

- Blood stasis due to *qi* stagnation.

- Stagnation of *qi* due to accumulation of blood in the interior.

- Simultaneous formation of both blood stasis and *qi* stagnation due to trauma by sprain and contusion.

Since the liver's dredging function plays a key role in the regulation of the functional activities of *qi*, stagnation of *qi* and blood stasis are closely connected to the physiological dysfunction of the liver. Additionally, since the heart is responsible for the circulation of blood, its physiological dysfunction leads first to blood stasis and then to stagnancy of *qi*, both marked by such symptoms as distending pain, ecchymosis, and abdominal mass.

Failure of *Qi* to Control Flow of Blood. Failure of *qi* to control the flow of blood is due to the deficient *qi* marked by various kinds of bleeding. Because *qi* is derived from the spleen, its dysfunction in transport causes deficient *qi*; in short, there is an inadequate production of *qi*. Since *qi* controls blood circulation, its deficiency promotes bleeding; in this case, *qi* is too weak to control the flow of blood. Finally, since the spleen dominates upward flow of *qi*, deficient *qi* in the middle-*jiao* and its sinking promotes the escape of blood from the lower part of the body, as is often seen in such symptoms as metrorrhagia and blood in the stool.

Exhaustion of *Qi* Resulting from Hemorrhage. Exhaustion of *qi* as a result of hemorrhage is a morbid state displayed as massive bleeding resulting in deficiency and exhaustion of both *qi* and blood. Massive blood loss can be the result of trauma or metrorrhagia and postpartum hemorrhage. Since blood is the carrier of *qi*, exhaustion of blood leads to the loss or exhaustion of *qi* (and blood). As a result, exhaustion of *qi* and blood promotes sudden severe functional failure of the human body.

Deficient *Qi* and Blood. The simultaneous deficient *qi* and blood is a morbid state resulting from either:

- The consumption of blood after protracted illness or loss of blood followed by consumption of *qi.*
- Decreased production of blood due to *qi* deficiency.

Clinically, this condition manifests as pale or yellowish complexion, shortness of breath, disinclination for talk, fatigue and weakness, emaciation, palpitation, insomnia, and/or numbness of the limbs.

Failure of *Qi* and Blood to Nourish Channels. Failure of *qi* and blood to nourish the channels refers to a morbid state of abnormal movement or abnormal sensation of the limbs, tendons, and muscles caused by the deficient *qi* and blood or the derangement of *qi* and blood.

The tendons, muscles, and skin depend on *qi* and blood for their nourishment. *Qi* and blood circulate through channels. If *qi* and blood are sufficient enough to interact on each other, tendons and muscles, well nourished, can function to facilitate movements of the limbs and the skin. Conversely, if the channels, tendons, muscles and skin are not properly nourished due to deficient *qi* and blood or derangement of *qi* and blood, then the following symptoms may result:

- Numbness of the limbs
- Paralysis of the limbs
- Itching and dryness of the skin
- Dry and scaly skin

7.5 Disturbance in Fluid Metabolism

Fluid metabolism is the process of constant production, distribution and excretion of body fluid. An imbalance between production and excretion results in insufficient body fluid due to reduced production, excessive consumption and excretion, or in such pathologic changes as fluid retention, stagnation, and overflow brought about by sluggish fluid circulation. Normal production, distribution and excretion of body fluid are inseparable from the following:

- Ascending-descending and incoming-outgoing movements of *qi* and its functional activities.
- Transporting and transforming functions of the spleen.
- Dispersing and descending function of the lungs.
- Water-regulating function of the kidneys.
- Clearance and regulation of the water passage by tri-*jiao.*

This condition produces pathological changes such as insufficient body fluid, retention of phlegm and accumulation of dampness.

Insufficient Body Fluid. Insufficient body fluid refers to a pathologic state marked by dryness and resulting from a failure of body fluid (which is insufficient in quantity) to moisten and nourish the *zang* organs, pores, skin and hairs. Insufficient body fluid is primarily caused by consumption of body fluid by:

- Pathogenic dryness-heat
- Disorders of the five emotions
- Profuse perspiration, vomiting, diarrhea, or loss of blood
- Excessive intake of drugs of acrid taste and drying effect

From the viewpoint of pathogenesis, insufficient body fluid is divided into two phases:

1. Impairment of *jin* (thin and clear body fluid)
2. Exhaustion of *ye* (thick body fluid)

Since *jin* is highly mobile, it is easily consumed and supplied. Manifestations of impaired *jin* include: profuse perspiration in hot weather, thirst due to high fever, and sunken eye and spasms due to severe vomiting, severe diarrhea, or diuresis.

On the contrary, *ye* is sluggish in motion and not easily consumed. Once consumed, it is not easily replenished. Clinical manifestations include:

- Exhaustion of *yin*-fluid or wind-stirring due to *yin* deficiency in the late stage of a febrile disease or after prolonged illness
- Reddish tongue with little or no coating
- Emaciation
- Withered muscles and skin
- Dryness of the hair on limbs
- Cramps or involuntary movement of the limbs

Impairment of *jin* is not necessarily accompanied by the exhaustion of *ye*. Yet *ye* depletion is certainly to be followed by impairment of *jin*. From the above it follows that impairment of *jin* is a gradual start of exhaustion of *ye*, which, in turn, is the climax of impairment of *jin*.

Disturbance in Distribution and Discharge of Body Fluid. Distribution and discharge of body fluid are the two important links in metabolizing body fluids, and functional disturbance of these links may lead to fluid retention, which is then transformed into phlegm and dampness.

Distribution. A disturbance in distribution of body fluid leads to sluggish circulation and localized accumulation of dampness, which is transformed into phlegm retention. The factors contributing to this disturbance are numerous; however, it results mainly from dysfunction of the lungs, spleen and liver and obstruction of tri-*jiao* as passageway of these factors.

Discharge. Disturbance in the discharge of body fluid results in edema and is due to weakened ability of internal organs to transform fluid into sweat and urine. Body fluid depends on the lungs' dispersing and descending function for its transformation into sweat to be excreted and on the functioning of kidney-*qi* for its transformation into urine to be discharged. Therefore, discharge disturbance of body fluid results mainly from functional disturbance of the lungs and kidneys. Functional disturbance of the kidneys and disturbance in formation and discharge of urine eventually leads to water retention, thus forming edema.

Water Retention Leading to Stagnation of *Qi.* Water retention leading to the stagnation of *qi* refers to the pathologic state characterized by stagnation of *qi* due to metabolic disturbance of body fluid, including retention of water and phlegm. Water retention and stagnation of *qi* can be the cause or effect of each other. For example, water retention in the lungs impedes the functional activities of lung-*qi*, which manifests as fullness of the chest, cough, and asthma. On the other hand, water retention in the heart obstructs heart-*qi* and inhibits heart-*yang*, which manifests as palpitation pain in the heart. Likewise, water retention in the middle-*jiao* may hinder functional activities of the spleen and stomach, leading to failure of clear *qi* to ascend and of turbid *qi* to descend, which manifests as dizziness, fatigue, distension and fullness in the epigastrium, and anorexia.

Exhaustion of *Qi* Resulting from Depletion of Body Fluid. The exhaustion of *qi* resulting from the depletion of body fluid is a morbid state indicating depletion of *qi* as a result of a massive loss/consumption of body fluid, commonly caused by high fever, profuse perspiration, severe vomiting, or diarrhea. Since body fluid and blood are the carriers of *qi*, loss of body fluid deprives *qi* of its carrier and thus *qi* is exhausted externally as well.

Blood Inadequacy Due to Exhaustion of Body Fluid. The inadequacy of blood due to exhaustion of body fluid refers to the pathologic state of extreme exhaustion of body fluid that produces heat of the deficiency-type and wind. The resulting conditions include:
- Impairment of body fluid by high fever.
- Consumption of body fluid by fever in chronic consumptive diseases.

- Loss of blood and fluid heat of *yin* deficiency type inside the body.

This condition manifests as restlessness or dysphoria with feverish sensation in the chest, palms and soles; dryness of the nose and throat; and itchy, scaly, and dry skin.

Blood Stasis Due to Loss of Body Fluid. Loss of body fluid—due to high fever, burns, vomiting, diarrhea and profuse perspiration—causes sluggish blood circulation, which leads to blood stasis. Clinical manifestations include insufficient body fluid, purplish tongue, and skin eruption.

7.6 FIVE ENDOGENOUS PATHOGENS

The Five Endogenous Pathogens are actually the five pathologic changes—namely, wind-transformation, cold-transformation, dampness-transformation, dryness-transformation, and fire-transformation—resulting from a disturbance in physiological functions of *qi*, blood, body fluid, and the *zang-fu* organs. (Since the transformation occurs inside the body, they are also referred to as endogenous wind, endogenous cold, endogenous dampness, endogenous dryness, and endogenous fire, respectively.) They are, therefore, five comprehensive changes of pathogenesis rather than pathogenic factors.

Endogenous Wind. Endogenous wind, also referred to as wind stirring inside the body, is a morbid condition caused by hyperactivity and adverse flow of *yang-qi*. During the course of a disease, hyperactivity of *yang* transforms into wind-syndrome due to excess of *yang* or inability of insufficient *yin* to inhibit hyperactive *yang*. It is marked by pathological changes such as tremors, dizziness, and convulsions.

Endogenous wind is often called liver-wind or liver-wind stirring inside the body because its occurrence is closely related to the liver. Wind syndrome of this type may be caused by hyperactivity of liver-*yang*, extreme heat, deficient *yin*, or deficient blood.

Wind Syndrome Due to Hyperactivity of Liver-*yang*. This syndrome is caused by deficient liver-*yin* and kidney-*yin* due to their impairment by disorders of the five emotions or overstrain, lending to exuberant liver-*yang* and manifested as tremors, dizziness, dry mouth, distorted eyes, and even sudden fainting or syncope accompanied by cold limbs.

Occurrence of Wind Syndrome in the Case of Extreme Heat. This syndrome is caused by an overabundance of pathogenic heat that consumes body fluid, impairs blood and the liver channel, and leads to malnutrition of the muscles and tendons. Its clinical manifestations are convulsion, hyperphoria accompanied by high fever, coma, and delirium, often seen in the climax of a febrile disease.

Wind Syndrome Due to *Yin* Deficiency. Wind syndrome due to *yin* deficiency is caused by the depletion of *yin*-fluid, which leads to malnutrition of the tendons and vessels and manifests as muscular twitching and cramping, as well as involuntary movement of the limbs. Note that the pathogenesis and clinical manifestations of this type of wind syndrome differ from that those that result from wind syndrome due to hyperactivity of liver-*yang* or to extreme heat.

Wind Syndrome Due to Blood Deficiency. Wind syndrome due to blood deficiency indicates endopathic wind of deficiency type stirring up inside and brought about by failure of insufficient liver blood to nourish tendons and vessels. It also results from failure of blood to nourish collaterals because of decreased blood production, blood loss, or protracted illness. Its clinical manifestations are: numbness of the limbs, and muscular constriction.

Wind Syndrome Due to Blood Inadequacy. Wind syndrome due to blood inadequacy is caused by:

- The depletion of body fluid and insufficient blood
- Blood consumption by protracted illness
- Insufficient blood and essence in older people
- Decreased production of blood due to chronic malnutrition
- Disturbance in blood production due to blood stasis

Its clinical manifestations are dry and/or scaly skin accompanied by itching.

Endogenous Cold. Endogenous cold is a morbid condition of internal cold or excess of *yin*-cold due to deficient *yang-qi* and its weakened warming function. Deficient *yang* results in relatively excessive *yin*, leading to internal cold and manifested as insufficient *yang*-heat, e.g., cold limbs, vascular spasm, and sluggish blood circulation. Since the kidneys are the root of *yang-qi*, deficient kidney-*yang* plays a key role in the production of internal cold. Deficient *yang-qi* reduces functional activities of *qi* and thus results in the accumulation of pathologic products of *yin*-cold type, such as water and phlegm, manifested as frequent copious urination, diarrhea, and edema.

Endogenous Dampness. Endogenous dampness indicates the morbid condition of water and phlegm retention within the body. It is caused by a disturbance of the spleen's transporting and distributing function. Since the spleen transports and transforms water, its dysfunction in transport is a leading cause of turbid dampness in the interior.

Therefore, this syndrome is also known as endogenous dampness due to deficient spleen.

Impairment of the spleen and stomach leads to functional disturbance in water transport and distribution and to retention of dampness, water, and phlegm. This, in turn, is likely to block spleen-*yang* and the middle-*jiao* thus aggravating the disturbance of the spleen's transporting function…which produces more dampness which further blocks spleen-*yang* and the middle-*jiao*; this cause-and-effect process forms a vicious cycle. In addition, when dampness blocks the middle-*jiao*, the symptoms include abdominal distention; poor appetite; greasy taste in the mouth; and thick, greasy tongue fur.

Endogenous Dryness. Endogenous dryness is a morbid condition characterized by insufficient body fluid, which thus fails to adequately moisten the *zang-fu* organs, tissues and pores. Insufficient body fluid results from:

- Impairment of *yin*
- Consumption of body fluid by protracted illness
- Pathogenic heat
- Profuse perspiration, severe vomiting, severe diarrhea, loss of blood or loss of essence of life

Insufficient body fluids—and thus endogenous dryness—leads to failure to irrigate the *zang-fu* organs internally and to moisten striae of skin and outer openings externally. This condition manifests as dryness and lack of luster of the skin; desquamation; cracked, dry mouth and throat; parched lips; dryness of the tongue; constipation, and scanty dark urine. Endogenous dryness is commonly seen in the lungs, stomach, and large intestine. In addition to the symptoms mentioned above, additional symptoms may be exhibited as follows:

- When lung-dryness is the primary symptom: dry cough without sputum or even hemoptysis.
- When stomach-dryness is the main symptom: reddened tongue without fur.
- When intestine-dryness is the main symptom: constipation.

Endogenous Heat. Endogenous heat, also known as pathogenic fire accumulated in the interior, is a pathologic state characterized by invasion of interior by pathogenic fire or hyperfunction due to:

- An excess of *yang*
- Hyperactivity of *yang* due to *yin* deficiency
- Stagnation of *qi* and blood
- Accumulation of pathogenic factors inside the body

The pathogeneses of endogenous heat may be summarized as follows:

1. Hyperfunction of *yang-qi* produces interior fire. This is what is known as "fire resulting from overabundance of *qi*." Hyperactivity of *yang-qi* gives rise to increased consumption of materials, thereby leading to the consumption of *yin*-fluid. This pathological hyperactivity of *yang-qi* is referred to as *zhuanghuo*.

2. Accumulation of pathogenic factors produces interior fire. Sometimes, any of the six pathogenic factors, i.e., wind, cold, summer-heat, dampness, dryness and fire, accumulate to produce interior heat. For example, cold accumulates and is transformed into fire; so does dampness. Other times, pathologic products of the body, such as phlegm, stagnated blood, malnutrition due to parasitic infestation, and food retention, accumulate and transform into fire. Its mechanism lies in that all of the above factors can lead to stagnation of *yang-qi*, thus producing heat to be transformed into fire.

3. The five emotions in excess produce endogenous heat. In other words, emotional upsets result in stagnation of *qi* and produce interior heat. For instance, stagnation of liver-*qi* gives rise to liver-fire.

4. Consumption of *yin*-essence gives rise to hyperactivity of *yang* and thus causes fire of the deficiency type to accumulate in the interior of the body.

7.7 PATHOGENESIS OF THE *ZANG-FU* ORGANS

A disease, whether due to external infection or internal injury, is likely to lead to disturbance in physiological functions of the *zang-fu* organs and dysfunction of *yin-yang*, *qi* and the blood of *zang-fu* organs. This syndrome, therefore, indicates the intrinsic mechanism of a disturbance in the normal physiological functions of the *zang-fu* organs.

Generally speaking, *yin* and *yang* of the *zang-fu* organs represent the functional state of physiological activities of *zang-fu* organs, (i.e., exciting or inhibiting, ascending or descending, dispersing or storing, etc.). Similarly, *qi* and blood of the *zang-fu* organs are the material basis of physiologic activities of various visceral organs Therefore there is a considerable difference between the imbalance of *yin* and *yang* of *zang-fu* organs and that of their *qi* and blood.

Relative Excessiveness of Heart-*yang*. This syndrome is indicative of the heart-fire, usually resulting from pathogenic heat, stagnation of phlegm-fire, and disorders of the five emotions. The main influence it has on the physiologic functions of the heart may be summarized as follows:

1. It disturbs the mind. Since *yang* is responsible for activity and ascent, exuberance of heart-*yang* may disturb the mind and cause excessive excitement that cannot be inhibited. This condition is marked clinically by palpitations, restlessness, insomnia, frequent dreams during sleep, polylogia, or even mania.

2. It causes blood-heat and swift blood flow. Exuberance of *yang* gives rise to heat, an excess of which, in turn, disturbs the heart's function in governing the blood and vessels. This, in turn, keeps blood circulating swiftly under the action of blood-heat and manifests as palpitations, rapid pulse, purplish red tongue with prickle-like fur—even bleeding.

3. It gives rise to flaring-up or moving-down of the heart-fire. As the tongue is the orifice of the heart, it can reflect the physio-logical and pathological states of the latter. If the heart-fire flames upward along the large collaterals, there will be such symptoms as ulceration of the mouth and tongue, burning pain at the tip of the tongue and dry mouth and nose.

   On the other hand, the heart is interiorly-exteriorly related to the small intestine. If the heart-fire moves downward along the channels to the small intestine, symptoms such as deep-colored urine and pain and burning sensation during urination occur.

Relative Deficient Heart-*yang*. Deficient *yang-qi* in the heart results from its constant consumption by chronic diseases. It can also be seen at the critical stage of an acute disease in exuberant pathogens overwhelm vital *qi* leading to sudden collapse of *yang-qi*. Its main effects on the physiological functions of the heart are as follows:

1. Reduced mental activities: When *yang-qi* is on the decline, it is unable to invigorate spirit, leading to weakened mental conscious-ness and thinking activities. As a result, one tends toward inhibition than to excitement. Clinically, there appears to be listlessness, weakened mental state, slow response, drowsiness, disinclination to talk, and low voice.

2. Blood stagnation due to cold. When heart-*yang* is insufficient, it can hardly promote blood circulation, and insufficient *yang* gives rise to cold. When cold attacks blood, blood circulation becomes slug-gish, leading to blood stasis or even stagnation of heart-blood and marked by:

- Chilliness and cold limbs
- Pale or dark purplish complexion
- Palpitations
- Oppressed feeling and stabbing pain in the chest
- Spontaneous perspiration and even profuse sweating
- *Yang* depletion
- Prostration syndrome
- Weak uneven pulse, slow pulse, rapid pulse or slow pulse with irregular intervals

Insufficient Heart-*yin*. Insufficient heart-*yin* (or deficient heart-*yin*) is caused mainly by consumption of heart-*yin* due to mental overstrain, improper care after chronic disease or emotional upsets, or exuberance of the heart-fire and liver-fire that impairs heart-*yin*. When heart-*yin* is insufficient, it fails to counterbalance *yang*, leading to relatively excessive heart-*yang* and fire of the deficiency type. When fire of the deficiency type disturbs the mind, there may appear such manifestations as irritability and insomnia. When fire of deficiency type attacks the blood vessels, there will be such symptoms as red tongue and small rapid pulse. When fire internally disturbs the body and body fluid is expelled together with *yang-qi*, *yin*-fluid cannot be kept within the body, marked by night sweating and other pathological manifestations.

Impairment of Heart-blood. Impairment or deficient heart-blood is often caused by blood loss, insufficient blood formation, or internal impairment by emotions. Deficient heart-blood leads to reduced blood circulation marked by a small, weak pulse and to neurosis due to inability to nourish the mind. This condition manifests as an inability to concentrate attention or even a state of trance. When blood is insufficient to nourish and retain heart-*yang*, the mind will not be nourished and mental activities are impaired. The result can be mental derangement, manifested as insomnia and dreaminess.

When the face is not properly nourished, then dim complexion and dryness of the tongue result. Additionally, failure of blood to nourish the heart causes symptoms such as palpitations or even panic.

Stagnation of Heart-blood. Stagnation of heart-blood (or blockage of the heart vessels) is marked by stagnation of blood in the heart vessels due to impeded blood circulation. The common causes of stagnation of heart-blood are:

1. Insufficient heart-*yang*, which gives rise to cold blood and impeded blood circulation.

2. Accumulation of phlegm, which impedes blood circulation.

3. Blood stasis, which obstructs the heart vessels and impedes blood circulation.

The disease is often induced or aggravated by overstrain, catching cold or emotional upsets. Due to obstruction of the heart vessels and impeded blood circulation, symptoms such as oppressed sensation and pain in the chest appear. In severe cases, stagnation and blockage of *qi* and blood manifests as severe palpitations, sudden attack of pain in the paracardium, cold limbs, deep-sited pulse and syncope after profuse sweating.

Deficient Lung-*qi*. Deficient lung-*qi* usually results from consumption of lung-*qi* by protracted illness or overstrain or from prolonged impairment of the lungs' dispersing and descending function. Insufficient lung-*qi* leads to weakened respiratory function and is marked by shortness of breath. When it affects distribution and metabolism of body fluid, it gives rise to phlegm retention and edema. When deficient lung-*qi* leads to obstruction of the defensive *qi*, the protective *yang-qi* is debilitated and skin is weakened, marked by spontaneous perspiration.

Impairment of the Lungs' Dispersing and Descending Function. This syndrome is usually caused by such factors as:

- Attack of the skin and the lungs by exogenous pathogens
- Obstruction of the pulmonary vessels by phlegm
- Upward invasion of the lungs by the hyperactive *qi* and fire of the liver
- Insufficient lung-*qi* or lung-*yin*

Generally speaking, exogenous pathogens often impair the lung's dispersing function, leading to obstruction of lung-*qi*, while internal injury affects the lungs' purifying and descending function, leading to their dysfunction. Nasal obstruction, chest stuffiness due to stagnation of the defensive *qi*, and obstruction of the skin all indicate the obstruction of lung-*qi*. If the lungs' dispersing function results from deficient lung-*qi*, it manifests as spontaneous perspiration due to lowered body resistance. The deficient lung-*yin* leads to failure of *yin* to retain *yang* and the consumption of body fluid following *yang* letting out, marked by night sweat. When the lungs' function of descending and purifying respiratory tract is impaired, abnormal rising of lung-*qi*, marked by cough with copious sputum and dyspnea appears.

Additionally, a weakened dispersing function and impairment of purifying and descending function of the lungs may actually influence each other in the pathologic process, either of which may cause abnormal rising of lung-*qi* and thus give rise to cough, disturbance in water metabolism, and edema.

Deficient Lung-*yin*. Deficiency or insufficient lung-*yin* is mainly due to impairment of the lungs by:

- Pathogenic dryness-heat or stagnation of phlegm-fire inside the body.
- Disorders of the five emotions in excess.
- Consumption of lung-*yin* by protracted cough.

Insufficient lung-*yin* results in:

- Decrease of the lungs' moistening function .
- Dryness syndrome.
- Abnormal rise of lung-*qi* due to disturbance of the lungs' ascending and descending function.
- Relative excess of *yang*, which gives rise to fire and heat of deficiency type.

Clinically, this condition manifests as dry cough with no sputum or with scanty sticky cheeks, dysphoria with feverish sensation in the chest, palms and soles, even blood-stained sputum resulting from damage of pulmonary vessels by fire of deficiency type.

Insufficient Spleen-*qi*. Insufficient spleen-*qi* (or *qi*-insufficient middle-*jiao*) is primarily caused by dysfunction of the spleen due to improper diet, congenital weak constitution, consumption after prolonged illness, or overstrain. Deficient spleen-*qi* results in impaired transporting-transforming function of the spleen, manifested as indigestion and tastelessness in the mouth. Similarly, deficient spleen itself leads to impairment of its function in sending up essential substances. This, in turn, affects the function of the stomach to send digested food downward, manifested in the upper part of the body as dizziness, in the middle part as distension in epigastrium, and in the lower part as loose stool and diarrhea. Dysfunction of the spleen due to its deficiency deprives *qi* and blood of their source, of growth and development, leading to systemic insufficient *qi* and blood. Moreover, deficient spleen also impairs its function in governing blood, manifested by blood loss. Finally, deficient spleen-*qi* also weakens its lifting function or even causes its collapse, manifested by prolapse of rectum due to lingering diarrhea and ptosis of internal organs.

Deficient Spleen-*yang*. Deficient spleen-*yang* is a morbid state further deteriorated by deficient spleen-*qi* and resulting from a disturbance of the spleen's warming function due to the decline of the fire from the gate of life. Deficient spleen-*yang* leads to endogenous cold of the insufficiency type and manifests as cold-type pain of the abdomen, diarrhea with undigested food in stool, and diarrhea before dawn. In addition, this condition also impairs the transporting and transforming function of the spleen, resulting in retention of phlegm and edema.

Insufficient Spleen-*yin*. Insufficient spleen-*yin* is mainly caused by consumption of body fluid and results from dysfunction of the spleen due to deficient spleen-*qi*. As a result of impairment of the spleen's transporting and transforming function, symptoms such as abdominal distention, loose stool, and indigestion may appear. As a result of insufficient body fluid, dry mouth and tongue and reddish tongue with little fur are common symptoms. Insufficient spleen-*yin* also results in dysfunction of the stomach, which causes the stomach-*qi* to fail to descend and to its adverse rising, marked by retching and hiccups.

Stagnation of Liver-*qi*. Stagnation of liver-*qi* is caused by sluggish functional activities of liver-*qi* due to dysfunction of the liver and resulting from emotional upset or depression. In the affected area, distending pain (e.g., bilateral hypochondriac fullness or pain in the right hypochondrium) appears. If stagnation of *qi* combines with that of phlegm or blood, the affected area displays lumps. These lumps manifest in the upper part as goiter and globus hystericus; in the middle part as lumps with distending pain in the breast, in the lower part as lower abdominal pain and distending pain in the testes. Moreover, stagnation of liver-*qi* and its transverse invasion of the stomach lead to adverse rising of stomach-*qi* and manifests as belching and acid regurgitation. When transverse invasion of the spleen by the hyperactive liver-*qi* occurs, diarrhea with pain occurs as a result.

Flaming Up of the Liver-Fire. This syndrome is created by the upward movement of the liver-fire, which is transformed either from the depressed liver-*qi* by violent rage that impairs the liver or from the five emotions in excess. As a result of extreme hyperfunction of liver-*yang*, there may appear such symptoms as distention of the head, headache, flushed face, congested eyes, irritability, excitability, and sudden attack of tinnitus or deafness. Excessive rising of liver-*qi* activates the stagnated fire, which is likely to impair *yin*-blood and lead to *yin* deficiency and hyperactivity of fire. If the liver-fire impairs the channels and vessels of the lungs and stomach, excessive rise of *qi* and fire may lead to stagnation of both *qi* and blood in the upper part of the body, resulting in syncope due to emotional upset.

Insufficient Liver-blood. Insufficient liver-blood is caused by excessive blood loss, consumption of blood, or weakened ability of the spleen and stomach to produce blood from protracted illness. Since the liver is an organ that stores blood, it is generally the first to be affected by an insufficient blood supply. Deficient liver-blood leads to:
  • Malnutrition of tendons and vessels and manifests as numbness of the limbs.
  • Restricted flexion and extension of joints.
  • Poor supply of blood to the head and eyes.

This condition manifests as dizziness, dim eyesight, eye dryness, blurred vision, and an uncomfortable feeling in the eyes as if there were foreign body in them. Moreover, deficient blood may also give rise to dryness-transformation leading to the stirring up of wind of the deficiency type, manifested by itching, chronic spasm of muscle due to trauma, or cramping.

Hyperactivity of Liver-*yang*. Hyperactivity of liver-*yang* is a morbid state characterized chiefly by abnormal ascending and floating action, hyperactivity, and adverse flow of the liver's *yang-qi* due to insufficient liver-*yin*, which is unable to counterbalance *yang*. It may also result from the deficient liver-*yin*, which is caused by the impairment of upward flow of *qi* and fire due to emotional disturbance. It may also develop into hyperactivity of *yang* due to *yin* deficiency. Since the liver and the kidneys have a common source, insufficient kidney-*yin*, which fails to nourish the liver, also leads to hyperactivity of liver-*yang* in the upper part of the body. This morbid condition often manifests itself by symptoms of an excess type (such as dizziness, tinnitus, flushed face, congested eyes, dim eyesight, irritability, and a taut, rapid pulse) and by those of deficiency type (such as lassitude in the loins and legs).

Up-Stirring of the Liver. Stirring up of the liver is caused by a variety of factors, such as exuberant pathogenic heat transformed into wind-syndrome, excessive liver-*yang* transformed into wind syndrome or massive consumption of *yin*-blood of the liver leading to malnutrition of tendons and vessels and stirring-up of endogenous wind of the deficiency type. The pathological manifestations of this condition are: tremor of the limbs, convulsion, muscular twitching, cramping and involuntary movement of the limbs.

Insufficient kidney-essence. Insufficient kidney-essence is mainly due to congenital deficiency essence reduced with age, consumption of essence by protracted illness or lack of proper care after birth. Insufficient kidney-essence may:

- Retard the growth and development of infants.
- Delay the beginning of menstruation.
- Impede the development and maturity of sexual glands at puberty.
- Lead to senility and hyposexuality among the middle-aged, marked by impotence and spermatorrhea.

If insufficient kidney-essence affects the sea of marrow (brain), clinical manifestations such as mental retardation and flaccidity of the legs appear.

"Unconsolidation" of Kidney-*qi*. The term "unconsolidation" refers to the inability to keep kidney-*qi* in tact, resulting in the random dispersion of kidney-*qi*. This syndrome is a morbid state mainly due to:

- Deficient kidney-essence in children.
- Decline of the kidney-essence in the aged.
- Chronic consumption of kidney-*qi* owing to early marriage or intemperance in sexual life.
- Protracted illness.

Unconsolidation of kidney-*qi* leads to inability to control defecation and urination, manifested as fecal and urinary incontinence and enuresis. When the kidneys malfunction, kidney-essence is easily lost, thus leading to seminal emission and spermatorrhea. This morbid state impairs the air-receiving function of the kidneys and dyspnea occurs even on slight exertion.

Deficient Kidney-*yin*. Deficient kidney-*yin* is a morbid condition chiefly due to consumption of the *yin*-fluid of internal organs and subsequent impairment of kidney-*yin* by protracted illness. It may also be attributed to blood and fluid loss or excessive intake of drugs for warming the kidneys to invigorate *yang* or to consumption of kidney-*yin* by intemperance in sexual life. Deficient kidney-*yin* gives rise to hyperactivity of kidney-*yang* leading to hyperactivity of fire and interior heat syndrome and marked by emaciation; dysphoria with feverish sensation in the chest, palms and soles; hectic fever; flushed cheeks; night sweats; reddened tongue with little fur; and thready, rapid pulse.

Insufficient Kidney-*yang*. It is a morbid condition mainly due to enduring deficient heart-*yang* and spleen-*yang*, which affect the kidneys and consume kidney-*yang*. It is also attributable to impairment of kidney-*yang* by intemperance in sexual life. Deficient kidney-*yang* gives rise to *yin*-cold in the interior, clinically manifested by obvious cold syndrome. For instance, it can impede the reproductive function, causing impotency and sterility due to cold sperm; it can also impair water metabolism and result in edema or a heart attach by retained fluid. Finally, as a result of deficient kidney-*yang*, the spleen is not properly warmed, leading to weakened transporting and transforming function of the spleen and marked by diarrhea with undigested food in stool or diarrhea before dawn.

Insufficient Stomach-*qi*. Insufficient stomach-*qi* is a morbid condition resulting chiefly by:

- Long-term improper diet
- Congenital weak constitution
- Instability to recover from a protracted illness

This condition weakens the ability of the stomach to receive and transform food and thereby manifests as poor appetite, tastelessness in the mouth, and anorexia. It also leads to dysfunction of the stomach in transporting food downward marked by fullness in epigastrium, belching, nausea, vomiting, and hiccups due to adverse rising of stomach-*qi*.

Deficient Stomach-*yin*. Deficient stomach-*yin* refers to exhaustion of fluid in the stomach due to consumption because of lingering pathogenic fever at the late stage of a febrile disease or because of a protracted illness. This condition leads to extreme dysfunction of the stomach in receiving and transforming food and manifests as anorexia, red and dry tongue, or even mirror-like tongue (tongue without fur). In addition, deficient stomach-*yin* leads to dysfunction of the stomach in transporting food downward, marked fullness in epigastrium, repeated nausea, and retching.

Stomach-cold. Stomach-cold is a morbid state due to impairment of stomach-*yang* resulting from excessive intake of cold and raw food, drugs of cold nature, or congenital insufficient *yang* complicated by an attack of pathogenic cold on the middle-*jiao*. Stomach-cold leads to sluggish functional activities of *qi* and contraction of meridians, often marked by severe epigastric pain that warmth relieves. It also leads to dysfunction of the stomach in transforming food into chyme, marked by indigestion.

Stomach-heat. Stomach-heat is mainly due to attack of the stomach by pathogenic heat—caused by an indulgence in alcoholic drinks; preference for hot, pungent food; and an excessive intake of food rich in fat. Stomach-heat is also caused by an accumulation of heat in the stomach transformed from stagnated *qi*, blood stasis, and retention of phlegm or food. Stomach heat gives rise to hyperfunction of the stomach and is marked by an unpleasant hungry sensation.

Exuberant stomach-heat consumes body fluid, resulting in accumulation of pathogenic dryness-heat and dysfunction of the stomach in transporting food downward, marked by bitter taste in the mouth, thirst, constipation, or deficient stomach-*yin*. When the fire transformed from the stomach-heat flares up, it leads to adverse rising of stomach-*qi*, marked by nausea and acid regurgitation. When the fire flares up along the channels, it gives rise to gingivitis or gingival hemorrhage. Furthermore when the fire impairs the stomach vessels, blood flows upward to produce hematemesis.

CHAPTER 8

Diagnostic Method

8.1 DIAGNOSTIC METHOD

The diagnostic method refers to the four basic techniques for diagnosis. They are: inspection auscultation, olfaction, interrogation and palpation. TCM holds that the human body is an organic whole whose component parts are physiologically interconnected and pathologically interactive. Therefore, local lesions affect the entire body and disorders of internal organs, in turn, manifest on the body's surface, especially on the five sense organs and the extremities. Diagnosticians use the four techniques to examine a disease's symptoms and signs, allowing them to determine the disease's causes, pathogenesis, and most effective treatment.

8.2 INSPECTION AND OBSERVATION

Inspection is a method of observing the patient's mental state, complexion, physical condition, and behavior to gain clinical data concerning the disease. All visible signs related to the disease are within the scope of inspection. Since the face and the tongue have close relation to the five *zang* organs and the six *fu* organs and since the vicissitudes of the *zang-fu* organs are most easily reflected by the appearance and color of these organs, they are the most common places for observation. Inspection of the superficial venules of the infant's index finger, as a special diagnostic method in pediatrics, is of great significance in the diagnosis of childhood diseases.

8.3 OBSERVATION OF VITALITY

To inspect a patient's vitality, one must observe the changes in the *zang-fu* organs. Vitality, a general term for life processes of the human body, is twofold:

1. Outward manifestations of all life activities

2. Thought and consciousness

Vitality cannot exist without a healthy physique; conversely, a diseased physique can certainty lead to abnormal vitality. As a result, the vicissitudes of vitality are an important mark of whether or not the physique is healthy. Vitality especially manifests in the eyes, and, therefore, observation of vitality is focused on the patient's eyes, as well as facial expression and behavior.

Possession of Vitality. Possession of vitality is a manifestation of abundant *qi*-blood of the *zang-fu*-organs, commonly seen in a healthy person. In a patient, it implies a mild illness without serious damage to the vital *qi*, often accompanied by a favorable prognosis. Its manifestations are: full consciousness, clear utterance, bright eyes, lustrous face, sharp response, natural posture, easy breath, fine-looking flesh, and regular urination and defecation. Among them, full consciousness and clear utterance result from sufficient vital essence of the heart; bright eyes, sharp response and natural posture from abundant vital essence of the liver and kidneys; and easy breath and fine-looking flesh from abundant vital essence of the spleen and lungs.

Loss of Vitality. When vital essence and *qi* in the *zang-fu* organs are impaired. In a patient, it indicates a very serious case. Its main manifestations are unconsciousness, apathetic expression and dull look in the eyes, lusterless complexion, sluggish response, faint breath, and emaciation. Among them, unconsciousness, apathetic expression, and lusterless complexion are caused by exhaustion of vital essence of the heart; a dull look in the eyes and sluggish response are caused by exhaustion of vital essence of the liver and kidneys; faint breath is caused by exhaustion of vital essence of the lungs; and emaciation by exhaustion of vital essence of the spleen.

Pseudo-vitality. Pseudo-vitality is the false appearance of symptom relief in a critically ill patient at his or her last breath. For example in a chronically or seriously ill patient, increased speech and bright eyes instead of a feeble voice and dull eyes; good appetite and raised food intake instead of original poor appetite; or flushing of zygomatic region—like wearing make-up—instead of original pale or sallow complexion. Because of the depleted *yin*-essence's inability to keep *yang* within the body, pseudo-vitality occurs; in short, *yin* and *yang* dissociate due to the outward floating of *yang*, which has lost its basis and its consumption of the remnants of the *yin*-essence.

8.4 OBSERVATION OF COMPLEXION

Observation of complexion refers to watching the color and luster of the patient's face. Color and luster are regarded as the outward manifestation of the ability of *qi*-blood in the *zang-fu* organs to nourish body surface. TCM holds that the complexion of a healthy person is shiny and lustrous, although it differs much in different races, natural endowment, and some physiological functions. The complexion of a patient in a morbid state is said to be sickly, which is characterized by:

- Darkness and lusterlessness.
- Excessive brightness and distinctness.
- Failure to correspond to appropriate seasons and relevant regions of the *zang-fu* organs in spite of its brightness and luster.

Physicians in ancient China classified the complexion as white, yellow, red, and blue, corresponding to different diseases respectively. Consequently, the face is the chief location for color observation.

White. The white complexion is a manifestation of deficient *qi* and blood and their poor supply to the face. A white complexion indicates deficiency syndrome, cold syndrome, and blood loss. It is mostly due to sluggish blood circulation resulting from:

- Insufficiency or the failure of *qi* to nourish the face.
- Deficient *qi* and blood.
- Sudden profuse bleeding causing depletion of the vessels.
- Contraction of the vessels invaded by pathogenic cold.

In general, a white or white-with-lusterlessness complexion is mostly attributed to insufficient *yang-qi*; a light white complexion is attributed to weakness of *qi*; a pale or sallow complexion is caused by a deficiency or loss of blood; and a pale complexion is accompanied by acute abdominal pain or shivers attributable to interior-cold syndrome.

Yellow. The yellow complexion is frequently related to a spleen disorder and is a manifestation of dysfunction of the spleen in transport, retention of water within the body, or deficient *qi* and blood. Specifically, a yellowish complexion with lusterlessness is attributable to deficient *qi* and blood; sallow and puffy face to inner retention of pathogenic dampness; and yellow-brown pigmentation of the skin of the whole body and sclera to jaundice, which is classified into two types: *yang* jaundice and *yin* jaundice. The former is characterized by bright yellow color like an orange peel, caused by steaming of damp-heat in the body; and the latter by dim yellow color like being smoked, resulting from the stagnation of cold-dampness.

A dark yellow complexion accompanied by expanded abdomen and venous engorgement is attributable to the disease tympanites. Additionally, infantile malnutrition is indicated by a sallow and swollen face, bluish-yellow complexion, or a yellow complexion with white cheeks, accompanied by the dried and withered hairs knotted like the ears of grain and abdominal dilation.

Red. A red complexion is due to the upward replenishment of the face with the *qi* and blood in their quick flow resulting from invasion of the pathogenic heat. Heat syndrome is of two types: excess-heat syndrome and deficiency-heat syndrome. The former is characterized by flushing on the entire face accompanied by thirst and dark urine. It is often seen in exogenous disease or febrile disease affecting *zang-fu* organs. The latter is characterized by flushed tender cheeks resulting from hyperactivity of fire due to a *yin* deficiency. In chronically or seriously ill patients, flushes or light red and white blotches appear on the face in gusts after the original pallor. This is known as floating *yang*, a critical syndrome marked by internal cold syndrome with external pseudo-heat symptoms and a failure of *yin* and *yang* to connect with each other.

Blue. The bluish complexion results from constriction of channels and stagnation of *qi* and blood due to invasion of the pathogenic cold. Moreover, stagnation of *qi* and blood leads to pain and malnutrition of the tendons and vessels and to convulsion and spasm. Therefore, the bluish complexion is a sign of cold syndrome, pain syndromes, blood stasis, and convulsion. The bluish color appears in different facial regions with different disorders. For example, with infantile convulsion or a tendency towards convulsion, the bluish color often appears between the eyebrows, on the bridge of the nose or around the lips. Bluish-purplish lips and bluish-gray face may be seen in patients with insufficient heart-*yang* and stagnation of heart-blood. A bluish face with flushed ears is mostly attributable to liver-fire; the bluish-red and lusterless-dark complexion to depressed fire and bluish complexion in women (accompanied by dysphoria with irritability, distending pain of the breast or irregular menstruation) to prolonged stagnation of liver-*qi*.

8.5 OBSERVATION OF BODILY FIGURE

The aim of observing the bodily figure is to see whether the patient is strong or weak; obese or thin; and to find out other conditions concerning the trunk, limbs, and body type. For instance, the strong body build implies sound internal organs and exuberance of *qi* and blood, while the weak body build denotes fragile internal organs and deficient *qi* and blood. Individuals of obese figure are liable to production of phlegm-dampness, apoplexy, and sudden syncope; and those of emaciated figure to physical cough due to deficiency or *yin* and hyperactivity of fire. Congenital malformation of the body is attributable to congenital defect, while its acquired deformity, such as the barrel chest due to prolonged cough and tympanites with a emaciated body, is frequently caused by disease. In terms of *yin* and *yang*, those of long and slender figure are known as persons with the constitution of *yang* hyperactivity, while those short and fat are persons with the constitution of *yin* hyperactivity. Those of moderate figure are said to have *yin* and *yang* in equilibrium.

8.6 OBSERVATION OF BEHAVIOR

Different diseases manifest themselves by specific behaviors. Therefore they may be diagnosed by inspecting the patient's posture, gesture and motion. As examples:

- A patient with dexterous limbs who is able to toss about in bed and often faces outward while lying, is commonly described as having excess syndromes of *yang*-heat.

- A patient with a heavy body who is unable to toss about in bed and often faces inward while lying is frequently thought of as having cold syndrome of *yang* deficiency.

- A patient lying on one's back with stretched legs who often takes his or her clothes and bedding off (with disgust toward fire) is believed most often to suffer from heat syndrome.

- A patient sitting with one's chin up and who displays dyspnea with abundant expectoration is known to have an accumulation of phlegm-dampness in the lungs.

- A patient sitting with a hung head and who experiences shortness of breath and reluctance to speak is experiencing insufficient lung-*qi* and kidney-*qi*.

- A patient sitting with inability to lie flat and experiencing dyspnea due to reversed flow of *qi* is known to have an upward attack of heart-*yang* by retained fluid due to the kidney disorder.

Additionally, cough with dyspnea and an inability to lie flat due to latent fluid-retention within the lungs usually occurs in autumn and winter while muscular tremors of the body are mostly seen when wind syndrome is present.

8.7 OBSERVATION OF THE HEAD AND HAIR

An oversized or undersized skull in children is due generally to natural endowment, deficient kidney-essence, or congenital hydrocephalus. Severe vomiting and diarrhea, deficient *qi* and blood, or an inherent defect may cause a sunken fontanel in infants. A protruding fontanel may result from the upward attack of the brain by pathogenic heat. Involuntary shaking of the head is primarily promoted by wind syndrome or malnutrition of the brain due to deficient *qi* and blood. Dense black hairs with luster is an indication of adequacy of vital essence; a few yellow hairs with dryness and withering is mostly seen after a serious disease. Sudden and extensive loss of hair is usually caused by blood-heat with an invasion of wind. Sparse hair patterns in teenagers is attributable to a kidney deficiency or blood-heat and the withered hair knotted like the ears of grain in children is a sign of infantile malnutrition

8.8 OBSERVATION OF THE EYES

Bright eyes indicate the possession of vitality and are easy to cure even when they are diseased, while lusterless and dull eyes suggest loss of vitality and are difficult to cure when diseased. Persons with flaring heart-fire often have flushed canthi and those with flaring lung-fire, hyperemia of bulbar conjunctive. Yellow sclera is largely due to retention of damp-heat in the interior; exophthalmous to flaming of the liver-fire; marginal blepharitis to accumulation of damp-heat in the spleen; and red and swollen eyes with burning pain to the wind-heat of the liver channel. Slight puffiness of eyelids is seen probably in the early stage of edema and atrophy of eyeball in the depletion of the vital essence.

8.9 OBSERVATION OF THE EARS

Observation of the ear, the specific orifice of the kidneys, refers mainly to inspection of its color, shape, and changes of its excretion. For instance, a thin and withered auricle is due to deficient kidney-essence and a dried and sallow auricle to the depletion of kidney-*yin* as seen in the later stage of febrile disease. The red collateral at the back of the auricle, is often considered as a premonitory symptom of measles. Scaly and dry helix is seen in blood stasis formed in a protracted disease or in acute appendicitis. Profuse blocking of the external acoustic meatus is known as ceruminosis and pus flowing in the ear (yellow, white or reddish in color) as otopysis or otitis media suppurative, resulting mostly from the upward invasion of wind-heat or damp-heat in the liver and gallbladder.

8.10 OBSERVATION OF THE NOSE

The nose serves as the window of the lungs. A red and swollen nose with sores is a sign of blood-heat. A stuffy nose due to a nasal polyp is attributable to extreme heat in the lungs or stagnation of wind-dampness. When the apex of the nose is flushed with acne—named rosacea— the spleen and stomach fill with pathogenic heat that spreads to the blood stream. An ulcerative bridge of the nose often indicates syphilis, and a sunken bridge of the nose accompanied by sparse eyebrows indicates leprosy. When the nares flare, excessive lung-heat is present. An extreme case of near-death from lung-*qi* exhaustion is signaled by flared nares, dyspnea, and sweating over a prolonged period of time.

8.11 OBSERVATION OF THE LIPS

Ruddy and lustrous lips indicate sufficient stomach-*qi* and a balance between *qi* and blood. Pathologically, light white lips are often due to loss of blood, which promotes malnutrition of the lips; deep red lips to excess-heat; cherry-like red lips to gas poisoning; bluish-purplish lips to stagnancy of *qi* and blood; dry and cracked lips to consumption of body fluid and involuntary salivation to insufficient spleen with overabundance of dampness or stomach-heat as seen in patients with apoplexy. Itchy, red and swollen lips with liquid oozing out from the cleft lip is called exfoliative inflammation of lips resulting from the upward attack of the pathogenic fire in *yangming* channel. The hard tender lip nodule that is as big as a silkworm cocoon is caused by the spread of phlegm-fire in the stomach to the lips.

8.12 OBSERVATION OF THE TEETH

Observations are made mainly to examine the luster, color and shape of the teeth and gums. Spotlessly white and moist teeth suggest plenty of body fluid; dry teeth, the consumption of body fluid due to excessive heat in the stomach; and extremely dry and lusterless teeth, the exhaustion of kidney-*yin*. As to the motility of the teeth, lockjaw indicates the obstruction of collaterals by wind-phlegm or occurrence of wind syndrome in the case of extreme heat. Likewise, the grinding of teeth during sleep indicates indigestion or malnutrition due to parasitic infestation. Loose and sparse teeth with exposure of the tooth root suggest the kidney deficiency.

In the case of gums, pale color indicates deficient blood; red and swollen gums (or inflammation of gums), flaring up of the stomach-fire; bluish lines appearing on the edges of the gums, lead poisoning; bleeding from red, swollen, and painful gums, impairment of collaterals due to the stomach-heat; and slightly puffy gums without redness and pain, deficient *qi* or deficient *yin*.

8.13 OBSERVATION OF THE THROAT

The disorders of the lungs, stomach, and kidneys may be reflected on the throat, observation of which aims chiefly at finding out whether there are redness, swelling, and/or a white membrane and a liquid secretion on the pharynx and larynx. As examples:

- Red, swollen and painful throat, sometimes accompanied by ulceration with pus, indicates tonsillitis due mostly to excessive pathogenic heat in the lungs and stomach.
- Reddish, slightly swollen and painful throat indicates hyperactivity of fire due to *yin* deficiency.
- Light red and slightly painful throat without swelling but susceptible to repeated attacks indicates deficient *qi* and *yin*.
- Loose and thick pseudo-membrane on the throat, especially if it is easily wiped out, most likely suggests stomach-heat
- Tough pseudo-membrane that is difficult to wipe out and which bleeds easily if forcedly stripped off indicates diphtheria due to excessive pathogenic heat in the lungs and stomach.
- Red and prominently swollen throat with the sensation of fluid wave suggests the formation of pus.
- Yellow and thick pus in the throat is frequently attributed to excess-heat.
- Thin and filthy pus in the throat is due to degeneration of vital *qi*.

8.14 OBSERVATION OF THE SKIN

The skin is most closely related to the lungs. When heart-fire and pathogenic wind-heat invade the blood, bright paint-like red skin is seen as in erysipelas. Red and swollen lower limbs indicate the downward flow of damp-heat; and the yellow-brown pigmentation of the skin can be seen in jaundice. Moist and lustrous skin suggests plenty of body fluid in the lungs, but on the contrary, dry skin with shedding of the vellus hairs indicates inadequate body fluid. Scaly and dry skin results mainly from blood stasis or formation of large carbuncle. Swelling of the whole body is described as edema, while only swelling of the abdomen, as abdominal distension.

Observation of Skin Eruption. Skin eruptions are commonly seen in patients with exogenous febrile diseases. The red discolored patch on the skin is known as macula by the outward dispersion of the pathogenic heat in the lungs and stomach from the muscles. The red and millet-like spots located above the skin are known as papula caused by outward dispersion of the pathogenic heat in the lungs and stomach from the skin. Ruddy and lustrous rashes distributed evenly indicate favorable prognosis; deep red ones, overabundance of the noxious heat; the dark purple ones, extreme noxious heat with large consumption of *yin* fluid; the light red or light purple ones, deficient *qi* and blood or decline of *yang-qi*. The scattered and thin rashes are seen in mild and shallow illness, while the dense and thick ones, in severe and deep disease. In addition rashes uneven in density or quickly disappearing are generally regarded as the critical symptom due to insufficient vital *qi* and pathogen invasion of the interior of the body.

Observation of the Miliaria Alba. The miliaria alba is a crystalline vesicle, protruding from the skin, oozing watery fluid after being broken and largely distributed over the skin of the neck, chest, and nape. It is mostly seen in patients suffering from the disease of summerheat and dampness and the damp-warm syndrome, both caused by damp stagnation on body surface with impeded perspiration. Therefore, miliaria alba is referred to as a manifestation of outward flow of the stagnated dampness. In morbid condition, the plump-eared miliaria, whitish in color and small in size, is called crystalline miliaria suggesting a favorable prognosis because of the abundance of vital *qi*. Conversely, the shrivelled miliaria without any fluid in it is called dried miliaria indicating an unfavorable prognosis of a serious case due to exhaustion of body fluid.

8.15 OBSERVATION OF THE TONGUE

The tongue, as the sprout of the heart, is related directly or indirectly to many *zang-fu* organs through the meridians. Therefore the vital essence of the *zang-fu* organs can nourish the tongue and any pathological changes of these organs may be reflected on the tongue. Observation of the tongue includes inspection of the tongue proper and the tongue fur, a layer of fur-like substance covering the surface of the tongue and formed by steaming of stomach-*qi*. By observing the tongue, a physician can predict the vicissitudes of vital *qi*, detect the depth of the location of illness, determine the nature of pathogenic factors, and infer the severity of disease. Hence, it plays an extremely important role in diagnosis in TCM.

Observation of the Tongue Proper. The tongue proper consists of muscles, vessels, channels, and collaterals in the tongue. Observation should include the mobility, color, size, and shape of the tongue proper.

The Pale Tongue. A tongue lighter than normal is known as pale tongue and results from the decline of *yang-qi*, leading to insufficient production of *yin*-blood or inability of blood to reach the tongue due to its diminished flow. In general, the pale and moist tongue with a puffy and tender body suggests cold syndrome due to insufficient *yang*, while the pale tongue with an emaciated body, deficient *qi* and blood.

The Red Tongue. A tongue that is a deeper red than normal is named the red tongue and indicates heat syndrome. It is a manifestation of fullness of collateral vessels with blood surge due to overabundance of heat. As examples:

- Bright red tongue with rough and prickly fur or with thick and yellowish fur suggests excess-heat syndrome.
- Red tip of the tongue indicates flaring-up of the heart-fire.
- Red margin and tip of the tongue with thin and yellowish fur is caused by the exogenous wind-heat.
- Bright red tongue with little fur, fissured tongue or the glossy tongue without any fur is a manifestation of heat syndrome of insufficiency type resulting from upward invasion of asthenic heat as a result of deficient liver- and kidney-*yin*.

The Crimson Tongue. A dark red color of the tongue proper is known as the crimson tongue. Indicating heat syndrome and blood stasis, it may be found in two types of disease: exogenous affection and endogenous injury.

- Crimson tongue or a tongue with a crimson spot in prickle-like fur (often seen in exogenous disease) is a manifestation of intrusion of the pathogenic heat into the blood system during a febrile disease and eruptions.
- Crimson tongue with little or no fur or with fissures is seen in endogenous disease suggesting hyperactivity of fire due to *yin* deficiency.
- Moist and crimson tongue coated with little fur suggests blood stasis.

The Purplish Tongue. A tongue purplish in color is seen in either cold or heat syndromes. The purplish tongue due to heat syndrome usually shows the crimson-purplish color with dryness resulting from the consumption of body fluid due to excessive heat and the stagnation of *qi* and blood. A purplish tongue seen in cold syndrome frequently shows light purple or bluish-purple color with moistness. Stagnancy of blood due to cold causes this, which further impairs *yang-qi*, thereby leading to retaining body fluid. That is why the tongue becomes moist. On the other hand, cold impairs channels, thus leading to sluggish blood flow or even stagnancy. That is why the tongue becomes light purple or bluish purple.

The Enlarged Tongue. The tongue body large in size or even filling up the whole mouth is called an enlarged or swollen tongue. As examples:

- Pale, puffy and tender tongue with moist fur and tooth marks on its margin is usually due to insufficient spleen-*yang* and accumulation of the phlegm-damp.
- Pink and corpulent tongue with yellow and greasy fur suggests damp-heat in the spleen and stomach.
- Bright red, swollen, and painful tongue is attributed to intense heat in the heart and spleen.
- Purplish and enlarged tongue indicates upward attack of the damp-heat with alcoholic toxicity.
- Puffy, bluish-purple, and lusterless tongue is due to stagnation of blood frequently seen in poisoning.

The Emaciated Tongue. A tongue smaller than normal in size is called emaciated tongue, a manifestation of failure of the collateral vessels in the tongue body to be replenished and nourished by the *qi* and blood and *yin* fluid. The emaciated tongue mainly indicates deficient *qi*, blood, or hyperactivity of fire due to deficient *yin*. Therefore, the emaciated, thin, and pale tongue is attributed mostly to deficient *qi* and blood, marked by dizziness, palpitation, sallow complexion, listlessness and lassitude. Conversely, the emaciated, dark red, and dry tongue indicates hyperactivity of fire due to deficiency and consumption of *yin*. This condition manifests as soreness and weakness in the loins and knees; dysphoria with feverish sensation in chest, palms and soles; dry mouth and throat; tidal fever with flushing of the zygomatic region and thready and rapid pulse.

The Fissured Tongue. The fissured tongue refers to fissures of different depths on the surface of the tongue and is a manifestation of failure of the tongue surface to be nourished and moistened with *yin*-blood. It suggests three morbid conditions, namely:

1. Consumption of *yin*-fluid due to excessive pathogenic heat.

2. Inability to supply nourishment due to blood deficiency.

3. Water retention within the body due to insufficient spleen-*qi.*

As examples:

- Dark red tongue with fissures most probably indicates consumption of body fluid due to intense heat or exhaustion of *yin* fluid.
- Pale tongue with fissures shows a blood deficiency.
- Pale, puffy, tender and fissured tongue with tooth marks on its margin suggests insufficient spleen function with retention of dampness, often accompanied by poor appetite, epigastric and abdominal fullness, and distension or loose stool.

The Indented Tongue. The tongue with tooth prints at its borders is known as the indented tongue and is a result of the pressure of dental coronae upon the puffy tongue. Therefore, the indented tongue often coexists with the puffy one. Since the tongue's puffiness is due to retention of water-damp within the tongue body caused by dysfunction of the spleen in transport, the indented tongue mainly indicates hypofunction of the spleen and excessive dampness.

- Pale and moist tongue with tooth prints at its borders usually suggests an excess of cold-dampness, whereas the pink tongue with tooth marks on its margin, hypofunction of the spleen or insufficient *qi.*

- The hyperplastic lingual papillae, protruding like thorns and causing a prickly sensation when they are palpated with finger are known as the prickled tongue, which is always due to an excess of the pathogenic heat, no matter where the pathogenic heat is and what stage the disease is in.

- Prickled tongue with scorching brown fur suggests excessive heat in the *qi* system.

- Crimson and prickled tongue without fur indicates consumption of *yin* fluid due to heat invading the blood system.

- The occurrence of prickles only on the tip of the tongue is often a result of heart-fire accompanied by irritability; thirst; scanty, dark urine; and rapid pulse.

- The occurrence of prickles on the margin of the tongue is a result of the fire of the liver and gallbladder, probably marked by flushed face with conjunctival congestion, bitter taste in the mouth, dry throat, and a wiry and rapid pulse

- Prickles on the middle of the tongue surface are a result of intense heat in the intestines and stomach, usually accompanied by such symptoms as thirst, constipation, and brown urine.

The Stiff Tongue. The rigid tongue body with inability to move freely is called the stiff tongue. As the tongue allows speech, the patient with a stiff tongue frequently suffers from dysphasia because exuberant exogenous heat consumes body fluid. This condition leads to malnutrition of the tongue if:

- It is caused by phlegm attacks the heart and if the mind fails to dominate the tongue.

- Hyperactive liver-*yang* obstructs the collaterals by windphlegm.

This morbid tongue syndrome is chiefly seen in apoplexy or pre-monitory symptoms of apoplexy due to an attack of the pericardium by excessive heat with body fluid involved and stagnation of phlegm in the interior. In summary:

- Deep red and stiff tongue usually indicates intense heat.
- Puffy and stiff tongue with the thick greasy fur often suggests phlegm-dampness.
- Pink or bluish-purplish tongue with rigidity is mostly seen in apoplexy.

The Flaccid Tongue. The weak tongue unable to protrude and curl is called flaccid tongue resulting mostly from failure of the tongue body to be nourished due to protracted deficient *qi* and blood or consumption of *yin* fluid. This morbid tongue is mainly produced by the following three pathogenic states:

1. Consumption of body fluid due to excessive heat.

2. Deficient *qi* and blood.

3. Extreme depletion of *yin* fluid.

As examples:

- Abruptly flabby and red-crimson tongue most probably indicates extremely intense pathogenic heat with impairment of *yin* fluid and is often associated with high fever, thirst, dry lips, scanty dark urine and rapid pulse.
- Gradually flabby and pale tongue suggests debility after protracted illness or extreme deficient *qi* and blood and is frequently accompanied by lassitude, weakness, dizziness, palpitation and pale and lusterless lips.
- Progressively flabby, dry and red tongue often associated with tinnitus and blurred vision and is most likely attributable to malnutrition of muscles and vessels due to deficient liver-*yin* and kidney-*yin.*

The Wagging Tongue. Caused by pathogenic heat in the heart and spleen, a wagging tongue moves incessantly. It is either a protruding tongue or a "played" tongue. A protruding tongue refers to frequent swelling of the tongue and the played tongue is characterized by:

- Slight protrusion of the tongue.
- Frequent drawing back of the tongue.
- Licking of the lips and corners of the mouth by the tongue.

Frequent protrusion of the tongue is usually seen in cases of attack of the heart by heat or exhaustion of the vital *qi*. Playing with the tongue is considered a sign of wind syndrome, mostly seen as a premonitory sign of convulsions or in infants with congenital hypoplasia, poor mental development, or mental retardation.

The Wry Tongue. A tongue turning to one side involuntarily while protruding is called the wry tongue. In most cases it is marked by an inclination of the anterior half of the tongue to either the left or the right side. This morbid tongue is mostly caused by obstruction of the collaterals on one side of the tongue body due to the liver-wind stirring-up inside the body with upward stagnation of phlegm or phlegm-blood stasis. Since the muscles on the affected side of the tongue are sluggish and weak and those on the healthy side contract normally, the tongue turns to the healthy side while protruding, indicating apoplexy or a premonitory sign of apoplexy. Pathologically, the purplish-red and wry tongue, associated with acute symptoms, most probably suggests convulsions due to intense liver-wind, while the reddish and wry tongue, accompanied by chronic symptoms, usually indicates hemiplegia due to apoplexy.

Observation of the Tongue Fur. The tongue fur is a layer of fur-like substance covering the surface of the tongue and formed under the steaming action of stomach-*qi*. Normal fur, white in color and even in distribution is spread thinly on the surface of the tongue. It looks like it grows out from the tongue rather than lying on top of the tongue like grease. Unhealthy, morbid tongue fur results from exogenous pathogens or retention of phlegm and food inside the body.

Inspection of the tongue fur is mainly made by observing its color, moisture, thickness, appearance, and distribution in combination with observation of the tongue proper. Such inspection furnishes information about the condition of body fluids as well as the nature and location of pathogens.

White Fur. Whitish and thin fur is usually seen in an exterior syndrome or a cold syndrome. In the case of an exterior syndrome, the fur appears at the onset of an exogenous disease that has not yet transferred its pathogens to the interior of the body. In the case of cold syndrome, however, white and moist fur spreads over the tongue like a heaped, moist powder. This is because of exogenous filthy-turbid pathogens or excessive pathogenic heat in the body. It is often seen in pestilence of abscess of internal organs.

Similarly, white, dry, and rough fur is due to sudden onset of internal heat and swift consumption of body fluid. In this case, the white fur fails to transform into yellow fur (as is usual) because of rapid conversion of the epidemic febrile disease into heat. Hence, white, dry, and rough fur remains.

Yellow Fur. Yellow fur, resulting from steaming the pathogenic heat, chiefly indicates heat syndrome. The deeper the yellow of the tongue fur, the more intense the pathogenic heat. As examples:

- Light yellow and thin fur indicates invasion by exogenous wind-heat.
- Yellow, thick, and dry fur suggests consumption of body fluid due to the stomach-heat and is often associated with thirst and constipation.
- Dark yellow, dry, and cracked fur suggests extreme heat and is often seen in organ diseases.
- Yellow, thick, and greasy fur indicates damp-heat in the spleen and stomach or the accumulation of heat in the gastrointestinal tract.
- Pale tongue with yellowish and moist fur is frequently due to hypofunction of the spleen with retention of dampness.
- Light yellow, moist, and thick fur—known as turbid fur— is attributed to the accumulation of dampness.

Gray Fur. Gray fur indicates an interior syndrome, which may be cold or heat in nature. In general, gray and dry fur usually occurs in exogenous febrile disease and is marked by fever and dysphoria. It may be seen in patients with hyperactivity of fire due to deficient *yin*, probably accompanied by lassitude in the loins and knees; dysphoria with feverish sensation in the chest, palms and soles; emaciated appearance; dry throat; flushed cheeks and tidal fever.

A gray and moist fur, however, suggests accumulation of damp-phlegm or retention of cold-dampness in the interior of the body and is often associated with stuffiness and choking sensations in the chest and epigastrium, heaviness in the limbs, and fatigue.

Black Fur. Black fur usually appears in the critical stage of an epidemic febrile disease, indicating the interior syndrome, either cold or heat in nature. Black and dry fur, even with prickle-like coating, is a manifestation of extreme heat and exhaustion of body fluid, often accompanied by such symptoms as high fever, flushed face, thirst with preference for cold drink, constipation, dark urine, coma, and delirium. Black and moist fur, however, is attributable to extreme *yin*-cold syndromes and is associated with cold limbs, cold-pain in the epigastrium and abdomen, watery diarrhea with undigested food in the stool, and a deep and slow pulse.

Thickness of the Fur. Thin fur refers to a thin layer of coating through which the tongue body can be indistinctly seen. Conversely, thick fur refers to a thick layer of coating through which the tongue body cannot be seen at all. The former is formed by upward aggregation of body fluid on the tongue surface due to upward steaming of stomach-*qi*, and the latter by upward retention of phlegm-dampness and food-drink on the surface of the tongue due to rising up of stomach-*qi*. The former is mostly seen in a healthy person or a patient having an exterior syndrome with the fur left unchanged, while the latter, in most cases, suggests an interior syndrome due to retention of phlegm, dampness, and food in the gastrointestinal tract. Generally speaking, the thin fur indicates a mild disease, whereas thick fur a severe disease. Fur that grows thicker and thicker indicates an unfavorable prognosis since exuberant pathogens continue to aggravate a disease. On the contrary, fur that grows thinner and thinner suggests a favorable prognosis due to predominance of vital *qi* and gradual decline of the pathogen.

Moisture of the Fur. The amount of body fluid may be estimated by observing the moisture of the fur. Lustrous fur, coated with moderate moisture, is thought of as normal, indicating plentiful and regular distribution of body fluid. Fur that looks excessively moist is named glossy fur, suggesting upward overflow of the retained dampness along the channels due to insufficient *yang-qi*.

Conversely, dry fur is caused by:
- Consumption of body fluid due to intense heat.
- Consumption of *yin*-fluid or inability of body fluid to be transformed and transported due to insufficient *yang*.
- Failure of body fluid to reach up the tongue surface due to pathogenic dryness that impairs the lungs.

In some special circumstances, the dry fur may also be seen in dampness syndrome and the glossy fur in dryness syndrome. Additionally, fur with rough grains spreading over the tongue is known as rough fur, frequently seen in cases of consumption of body fluid due to excessive heat.

Greasy and Curdy Fur. Curdy fur is attributable to overabundance of *yang-qi*, whereas greasy fur is due to retention of pathogenic damp-ness in the interior and depression of *yang-qi*. Big, loose, and grain-like fur can sometimes look like bean curd heaped on the tongue surface. This symptom is called curdy fur, which usually results from the ascent of stale and turbid substances and pathogens in the stomach steamed by excessive *yang*-heat. It indicates retention of food in the gastrointestinal tract or stagnation of phlegm in the interior often seen in abscess of internal organs.

On the other hand, compact and little grain-like fur, thinner on the margin and thicker in the middle of the tongue surface and difficult to scrape off is named the greasy fur—like grease covering the tongue surface. It is a result of retention of pathogenic dampness in the interior and on the tongue due to depression of *yang-qi*, marked by dampness, phlegm, indigestion, and damp-heat.

Exfoliative Fur. Tongue fur that exfoliates partially or completely is known as exfoliative fur. In general, the exfoliative fur is formed as a result of impairment of both stomach-*qi* and stomach-*yin*, with which therefore, the exfoliative fur varies in shape. The change from the presence of fur to its absence is a manifestation of deficient *qi* and *yin* and gradual weakness of vital *qi*. On the contrary, the regeneration of a thin and white fur after being stripped off is regarded as favorable sign of conquest of pathogens by vital *qi* and gradual recovery of stomach-*qi*.

As examples:

- A furless tongue as smooth as a mirror is appropriately named a mirror-like tongue.
- The partly exfoliative fur only (with the center of the tongue surface coated) is called chicken heart-like fur.
- Exfoliating fur that looks like an interlocking map is known as a map-like tongue.
- Scanty and scattered fur on the tongue surface is called *lingua geographica*.

8.16 OBSERVATION OF DISCHARGES

Discharges includes secretions and excretions. Fluids secreted from the ears, nose, mouth and eyes are known as secretions, whereas waste materials eliminated from the body as excretions. Discharges actually include both secretions and excretions, namely, saliva, vomit, stool, urine, vaginal discharge, nasal discharge, and tears.

Observation of discharges aims chiefly at examining their changes in appearance, color, amount, and nature, so as to find out pathological changes of the *zang-fu* organs. Generally speaking, the clear and watery discharges indicate deficiency and cold syndromes, whereas the dark (or red) and thick discharges, heat and/or excess syndrome. In addition, the blackish discharges mingled with some lumps of objects are usually attributable to blood stasis.

Observation of the Sputum. The sputum is a pathological product formed in the course of water metabolism of the body, closely related to the lungs and spleen. The sputum can be classified as follows:

- Profuse, whitish and thin sputum easily expectorated is referred to as damp-phlegm resulting from fluid retention due to hypofunction of the spleen.

- Sputum that is whitish and dilute as froth is due to wind-phlegm caused by the body fluid's failure to disperse regularly because of an invasion of the exogenous wind-cold pathogens or deficiency syndrome of the lungs due to protracted illness.
- Yellowish, thick, and even lump-like sputum suggests heat-phlegm resulting from pathogenic heat's concentration of body fluid.
- White, clear, and dilute sputum that may be mixed with some black spots indicates cold-phlegm, which is due to impairment of *yang-qi* by the pathogenic cold.
- Scanty and viscid sputum difficult to be spit is due to dryness-phlegm brought about when pathogenic dryness damages the lungs.
- Sputum mixed with bright red blood indicates heat injury of the blood vessels.
- Stinking expectoration with thick or purulent pus-blood is seen in pulmonary abscess.

Observation of the Vomit. Vomit refers to phlegm and food coming out of the mouth because of the adverse rising of stomach-*qi*. Vomiting due to different causes can produce different kinds of vomit and different accompanying symptoms and signs.

As examples:

- Clear, thin, and odorless vomit pertains to the cold-type vomiting due to insufficient stomach-*yang*.
- Sour, foul, viscid, and thick vomit suggests heat-type vomiting due to invasion by pathogenic heat.
- Vomiting of thin and profuse fluid accompanied by dry mouth and aversion to drink results usually from phlegm-retention.
- Sour and fetid vomit mixed with undigested food indicates retention of food.
- Intermittent vomiting accompanied by hypochondriac distension and eructation is due to an attack of the stomach by hyperactive liver-*qi*.
- Vomiting bright red blood or dark purple mass mixed with food residues suggests accumulation of stomach-heat or attack of the stomach by the liver-fire.
- Vomit mixed with pus and blood generates from stomach abscess.

Observation of Stool. Abnormal color and nature of stool may reflect pathologic changes in the spleen, stomach and intestines, as well as cold syndrome or heat syndrome, deficiency syndrome or excess syndrome of a disease.

- Loose stool and diarrhea with undigested food are due to disturbance of the spleen by cold-dampness or insufficient *qi* of both the spleen and the stomach, bringing about their dysfunction in transportation and transformation and retention of body fluid in the intestines due to their failure to receive and transport food.

- Dark yellow, foul and sticky stool indicates accumulation of damp-heat in the intestines.

- Red-white mixed and mucous stool is brought about by dysentery due to accumulation of pathogenic damp-heat in the large intestine and its intrusion upon both *qi* and blood.

- Whitish stool with profuse pus indicates excessive damp-ness in the *qi* system.

- Bright red blood defecated before feces, called " nearby bleeding," is often seen in hemorrhage from hemorrhoids and anal fissure or hemalochezia due to impairment of the lung collaterals by pathogenic wind-heat.

- Dark purplish blood defecated following feces implies bleeding from a distant part due to weakness of the spleen and stomach.

Observation of Urine. Normal urine is a light yellowish fluid.

- Clear and copious urine accompanied by aversion to cold and cold limbs often pertains to cold syndrome due to impairment of *yang*.

- Urine mixed with bright red blood is caused by heat in the small intestine or impairment of the collaterals of the small intestine by the descending hyperactive heart-fire. Light red urine denotes the hyperactivity of fire due to *yin* deficiency. Urine mixed with blood is called stranguria complicated by hematuria.

- Cloudy urine like oil is often known as stranguria marked by chyluria.

- Urine mixed with sand-like or stonelike objects accompa-nied by burning pain in the urethra on micturition and urinary stuttering is often referred to as stranguria due to urinary stone.

8.17 OBSERVATION OF SUPERFICIAL VENULES OF AN INFANT'S INDEX FINGERS

The superficial venules of an infant's fingers refers to collateral vessels emerging on the palmar aspect of the index fingers of a child, which are the branches of the Lung channel of hand-*taiyin*. They may reflect the changes of *qi* and blood of the *zang-fu* organs. This method is mainly used in children under three years of age because their skin is tender, which makes the venules easily visible. Observation of the superficial venules includes observation of their color, location, and shape.

Normal superficial venules of the index finger are located near the transverse crease between the palm and the index finger and extends from the proximal to the outside of *fengguan* (wind-pass). Those superficial venules visible on the proximal, middle and distant segment of the infant's index finger are referred to as *qiguan* (*qi*-pass) and *mingguan* (life-pass).

Color of the Superficial Venules of the Fingers. The color of the venules may be described as red, purple, blue, black and pale.

- Bright-red venules usually indicate attack of exogenous pathogens such as wind and cold.
- Purplish-red venules indicate heat syndrome.
- Bluish venules indicate wind-syndrome or pain-syndrome.
- Bluish-purple or purplish-black venules denote a critical stage due to blockade of superficial venules and pale venules, deficient spleen.

Length of Superficial Venules of the Fingers. The length of the superficial venules of the fingers is directly related to affected regions. \

- Generally speaking, if the collateral venules are only visible at *fengguan*, it indicates that pathogens have invaded the collaterals and the disease is mild.
- When the collateral venules are dark in color and extend from *fengguan* to *qiguan* they denote that pathogens have invaded the channels and a serious disease ensues.
- the collateral venules are visible at *mingguan*, it implies that the pathogens have invaded the *zang-fu* organs and the condition is dangerous.
- If the collateral venules directly reach the tip of the index finger, this is known as superficial venule visible from *guan* to the nail of index finger and it indicates that a disease is critical and will most probably be followed by an unfavor-

able prognosis. In summary, the superficial venules emerging at *fengguan*, *qiguan*, and *mingguan* reflect conditions that may be mild, serious, or critical in nature respectively.

Emerging Degree of the Superficial Venules of the Fingers.
The ease at which the superficial venules may be seen reflect the depth of the location of a disease.

- Visible venules indicate an exterior syndrome. This is often seen in diseases due to exogenous pathogens.
- Invisible venules indicate an interior syndrome. Thin and light-colored venules often denote a deficiency syndrome.
- Thick and dark-colored venules, indicate an excess syndrome.

The thickness and color of skin and the type of build also affect the emerging degree of the superficial venules as well. For example, the venules are easily visible on those individuals with thin skin. An obese person presents deep venules while a thin person, superficial ones. Consequently diagnosis can only be made in combination with other clinical data.

8.18 AUSCULTATION AND OLFACTION

Auscultation and olfaction are the diagnostic methods of detecting the clinical status of a patient by listening to his voice, breathing, coughing, and smelling the odors of his secretions and excretions. According to traditional Chinese medicine, all of the sounds and odors from the human body, produced in the course of physiological and pathological activities of *zang-fu* organs, may reflect physiological and pathological changes. Listening consists of listening to the changes in the volume and depth of a patient's speech or voice, as well as abnormal sounds that may accompany coughing or vomiting. In order to determine the nature of a disease, smelling various odors of the patient's body is involved as well.

Listening to the Voice. The voice is produced by the coordinated activities of the larynx, epiglottis, tongue, lips, teeth, and nose—and by functional activities of vital *qi*. Since the lungs control the *qi* of the body, the kidneys regulate inspiration and the heart governs speech, the voice is most closely related to the organs mentioned above. Once normal activities of *qi* are affected, whether by exogenous pathogens or by internal injury, the vocal organs are affected and the voice is likely to become abnormal. As a result, listening to the voice can detect changes of internal organs and the body as a whole.

Listening to the Speech Sounds.

- A loud speech sound often indicates excess syndrome or heat syndrome.

- A low and faint speech sound or disinclination to talk usually denotes deficiency syndrome or cold syndrome.

- A low voice accompanied by a stuffy and running nose and chills without sweating are indicative of affection by exogenous wind-cold.

- A deep and indistinct voice associated with the feeling of oppression over the epigastrium and a heavy sensation of the limbs is caused by retention of pathogenic dampness.

- Moaning and screaming are seen in pain-syndrome.

- Hoarseness is due to invasion of the epiglottis by pathogens.

Listening to Breath. Since the lungs control respiration and the kidneys regulate inspiration, abnormal breathing is mainly related to the lungs and kidneys.

- Feeble breathing is called insufficient *qi* and is often due to deficient vital *qi* in both the lungs and kidneys.

- Strong coarse and loud breathing is called rude respiration and is brought about by accumulation of pathogenic heat in the lungs.

- Rapid shallow breathing or difficulty of respiration, is called dyspnea which is classified into an excess-type and a deficiency-type. The excess type refers to loud and coarse breathing with a comfortable sensation upon expiration. The deficiency-type refers to weak and low breathing.

- Paroxymal rapid respiration with wheezing is called asthma; and is characterized by breath that is shorter and quicker than that of normal people. It is often accompanied by a rapid breath without wheezing and an oppressive and stuffy sensation in the chest due to stagnation of liver-*qi*.

Listening to Cough. Cough is a manifestation of purifying and descending functions of the lungs leading to adverse rising of lung-*qi*. When listening to cough, focus attention on the sound of the cough and changes in amount, color, and quality of the sputum in order to differentiate between cold or heat syndrome and deficiency or excess syndrome.

- A deep and raucous cough is often thought of as excess syndrome.

- A weak and clear cough reflects a deficiency syndrome.

- A dry cough with little or no sputum and with difficulty in expectorating pertains to dry cough due to attack of the lungs by pathogenic dryness or dryness of the lungs because of deficient *yin*.
- A cough with copious whitish sputum easily expectorated is due to an accumulation of phlegm-dampness in the lungs.
- A deep cough with thick and yellowish sputum not easily expectorated is due to heat cough due to invasion of the lungs by pathogenic heat.

Additionally, a children's cough characterized by spasmodic parox-ysm and a wheezing sound is referred to as whooping cough.

Smelling Odors.

- Foul breath is due to indigestion or a dirty mouth.
- Belching with sour and fetid oder denotes food stagnancy.
- Sweat that smells of fish or mutton is caused by accumula-tion of damp-heat in the skin. *Fetid odor from nose, with continual turbid nose discharge is often indicative of sinusitis.
- Expectoration of foul sputum with pus and blood can indicate a lung abscess.
- Fetid stool pertains to heat syndrome while stinking stool to cold syndrome.
- Scanty, foul, and dark yellow urine frequently indicates damp-heat syndrome.
- A foul smell like the odor of rotten apple from the mouth is attributed to diabetes.

8.19 QUESTIONING

Questioning is the diagnostic method of asking patients or their relatives about their particular problem. This plays an important role in the four diagnostic methods. Through inquiring, doctors can know the patient's case history, subjective symptoms, family history, and thera-peutic measures that have already been taken. When questioning, a doctor must be amiable without upsetting the patient.

8.20 QUESTIONING ABOUT CHILLS AND FEVER

Generally speaking, a state of chills is a disorder due to pathogenic cold, which is chilly in nature, while fever is due to pathogenic heat, which is scorching in nature. When an imbalance of *yin* and *yang* occurs, an excess of *yang* leads to fever, whereas an excess of *yin* causes chills. Conversely an excess of *yang* due to *yin* deficiency can also cause fever and excess of *yin* due to *yang* deficiency can cause chills.

Chills and Fever.

- Serious chills accompanied by a slight fever is often seen in exterior wind-cold syndrome, in which the predominance of the chills is caused by stagnation of defensive *qi* due to invasion of pathogenic cold. Because cold is a kind of *yin* pathogen, it easily damages *yang-qi* and a slight fever occurs when the body's defensive *qi* attempts to combat the invading pathogens.

- A higher fever with slight chills is often seen in exterior wind-heat syndrome. At this time excess of *yang* due to *yang* pathogens gives rise to high fever. Defensive *qi*'s inability to warm the body surface results in slight chills.

- A low fever with aversion to wind and spontaneous perspiration are often found in exterior syndrome due to invasion by pathogenic wind. Wind can cause the striae of skin to have a slight stagnation of *yang-qi* on the superficies of the body.

Chills without Fever. Chills without fever is often a symptom indicating that the patient has a subjective aversion to cold but not to heat due to long-time insufficient *yang*. The sensation of chills is often due either to invasion of pathogenic cold on the skin of the body or to a direct attack on the *zang-fu* organs. If pathogenic cold invades the skin, the patient gets no relief from supplied warmth because the attacking pathogenic cold prevents the defensive *qi* from reaching the body's surface. Unlike an invasion of the skin, a direct attack of the *zang-fu* organs generates abdominal pain with a cold sensation and deep slow pulse.

If the chills are due to a protracted illness, they result from a loss of body heat due to insufficient *yang-qi*. Keeping the patient warm can prevent *yang-qi* from being consumed and, therefore, the chills are likely to subside.

Fever without Chills. Fever without chills suggests that the patient has an aversion to heat but not to cold. This pertains to interior heat syndrome resulting from excess of *yang* or hyperactivity of *yang* due to deficient *yin*.

- Persistent high fever is called sthenic fever. Such a fever results at a critical stage of interior heat-syndrome due to formation of heat by exogenous pathogens and the interior invasion of pathogenic wind-heat. It is often accompanied by excessive sweating and excessive thirst.

- An intermittent fever that attacks at regular intervals like the rise and fall of tidal water is called a tidal fever. Tidal fever in afternoon is mostly caused by an accumulation of dry-heat in the stomach and intestines.
- A prolonged low fever is caused by insufficient *qi* and *yin* or by stagnated heat in the liver channel.

Alternate Attacks of Chills and Fever. Alternate spells of chills and fever are caused by half exterior and half interior syndrome. It is often accompanied by bitter taste in the mouth, dry throat, and dizziness due to a lingering of the pathogens between the exterior and the interior and a conflict between the vital *qi* and the pathogens.

8.21 QUESTIONING ABOUT PERSPIRATION

Sweat originates from body fluid and comes out of the pores and is evaporated by *yang-qi*. Normal sweating moistens the skin and regulates both nutrient and defensive *qi*. Abnormal perspiration occurs due to the invasion of pathogens or deficient vital *qi* during the disease process. Since abnormal perspiration varies with the nature of the pathogens and the degree of deficient vital *qi*, questioning about perspiration may help the doctor to differentiate the type of syndrome that is occurring. When questioning about perspiration one should be concerned with the type, amount, color, and location of the sweating that is occurring.

Spontaneous Perspiration. Spontaneous sweating intensifies when the body is exerted. Deficient *qi* and *yang* that brings about a lower superficial resistance mostly cause this. The body then lets fluid out due to loose striae. Spontaneous perspiration is often accompanied by symptoms of *qi*-deficiency that include, faint breathing, lassitude, shortness of breath, and disinclination to talk. Symptoms that accompany spontaneous sweating because of *yang* deficiency include aversion to cold, cold limbs, and watery urine.

Night Sweats. Night sweats refers to sweating that occurs when a person is asleep but not while they are awake. Night sweats have two common causes. One is heat syndrome in the interior caused by a *yin* deficiency. During sleep defensive *qi* enters the interior of an individual and an overabundance of *yang*-heat steams the body fluids and it comes out as sweat. When the individual is awake, the sweating stops because defensive *qi* leaves for the superficies of the body.

Profuse Perspiration. Excessive sweating is seen in patients that have an overabundance of pathogenic heat or sudden collapse of *yang-qi*. High fever, profuse perspiration, thirst, flushed face, and full-large pulse characterize an overabundance of pathogenic heat. This results from the inward invasion and heat-transformation of exogenous pathogens or the intrusion of wind-heat into the interior of the body. A sudden collapse of *yang-qi* is characterized by profuse and cold sweating, pale complexion, cold limbs, and indistinct pulse and is often seen in critically ill patients.

Profuse perspiration with hot and viscous sweat, accompanied by high fever, restlessness thirst, and a thready rapid pulse usually indicates a critical condition known as *yin*-exhaustion.

Perspiration after Shivering. In a critically ill patient, sweating following sever chills involving the whole body is called perspiration after shivering. It is a turning point in the development of pathological changes within the body. When this phenomenon occurs, close attention should be paid to the changes in the disease's development. If the fever subsides after sweating and the pulse calms down, the patient tends to improve because the body's *vital qi* is overcoming the invading pathogens. If high fever persists after sweating and is accompanied by an irritability and swift pulse, the disease is likely to be aggravated because the invading pathogens overcome *vital qi*.

Perspiration on Forehead. Perspiration on the forehead can be caused by several different factors.

- By dampness that is stagnated in the middle-*jiao* and the inward retention of damp-heat steaming body fluid upwards. It is often accompanied by a heavy sensation in the head and limbs, epigastric distention, and a greasy fur coating on the tongue.

- Pathogenic heat may be stagnated in the upper-*jiao* and an overabundance of *yang-qi* can evaporate the body fluid upward to the forehead. This type of perspiration is usually accompanied by restlessness, thirst, and red tip of the tongue.

- Forehead perspiration can also result from the floating up of asthenic *yang* due to consumption of vital *qi* after a prolonged disease. Perspiration of this type is accompanied by oily sweat over the head, cold limbs, dyspnea, and feeble, rapid pulse.

Hemihidrosis. Sweating just from one side of the body, either right or left, upper or lower, is called hemihidrosis. This type of sweating indicates that the sweating side is in a healthy condition, while the side without sweating is affected. A blockage of the channels and an obstruction of nutrient *qi* and defensive *qi* cause this. The pathogenic agents contributing to it may be wind-phlegm, blood stasis phlegm, or wind-dampness and is often seen in patients with apoplexy, flaccidity syndrome, or paralysis.

Excessive sweating of the Palms and Soles. Excessive sweating of the palms and soles is considered an abnormal state. There are several possibilities that may cause this.

- Dysfunction of the spleen and stomach in transporting and transforming nutrients may lead to lateral seepage of body fluid to the extremities.
- The steaming of stagnated heat in the *yin* channels may cause this condition as well. This occurs because the channel of hand-*jueyin* and foot-*shaoyin* pass through the palm and sole respectively. Therefore, stagnation of heat in these two channels results in sweating of the palms and soles. Dry mouth and throat, constipation, dark urine, and a thready and rapid pulse usually accompany this.

8.22 QUESTIONING ABOUT PAIN

Deficient *qi* and blood or blockages of the channels will lead to pain, which is one of the most common clinical symptoms and can occur in any part of the body. There are two causes of pain.

1. Stagnant *qi* and blood due to blockages of the meridians cause it. In most cases, it is brought about by an invasion of exogenous pathogens, *qi* stagnancy and blood stasis, or coagulated phlegm, all of which lead to pain of an excess type.
2. It results from malnutrition of the *zang-fu* organs and tissues due to deficient *qi* and blood. This is pain of deficiency type. When questioning a patient about pain close attention should be paid to the nature, location, and intensity of the pain that the patient is experiencing.

Headache. The head is the confluence of all the *yang*-channels. In TCM the brain is referred to as the sea of marrow and is closely closely related to kidney-essence.

Either exogenous pathogens or internal injury may cause headache. Because of the different distributions of the channels in the head, affected channels can be detected according to the location of pain.

- An acute headache involving the nape and back that exposure to wind aggravates suggests an exogenous disease due to invasion of pathogenic wind-cold.
- A distending headache accompanied by a flushed complexion and conjunctival congestion is due to an exogenous attack of pathogenic wind-heat.

- A sensation of heaviness in the head that is accompanied by chills and fever is caused by an exogenous attack of pathogenic wind-dampness.

- A moderate intermittent headache that lasts a long time usually pertains to pain caused by internal injury.

- A lingering headache, aggravated by exertion, is caused by a *qi*-insufficiency.

- Pain accompanied by dizziness and a pale complexion is due to blood-deficiency.

- An empty sensation in the head and lassitude in the loins and knees is caused by kidney-deficiency, which, in turn, is caused by insufficient kidney-essence and inability of the brain to be nourished.

Chest Pain. Since the chest is the place where the heart and the lungs are located, pain in the chest is mostly related to these two organs.

- A choking pain in the chest that sometimes extends toward the back indicates chest bi-syndrome. Hypofunction of *yang* in the chest and retention of paroxysmal phlegm or stagnation or an obstruction of *qi* and blood in the heart channel cause this syndrome.

- Chest pain accompanied by a flushed face, high fever and a shortness of breath mostly indicates an excess syndrome and denotes deficient lung-*yin*. Tidal fever, night sweats, and expectoration of bloody sputum accompany it.

Hypochondriac Pain. Since the liver and gallbladder are situated in the hypochondriac region, hypochondriac pain is related to these two organs.

- Distending hypochondriac pain that is accompanied by irritability indicates a stagnation of liver-*qi*.

- A burning pain in this region that is accompanied by a flushed face and pinkeye implies an accumulation of liver-fire.

- Hypochondriac and costal distending pain that accompanies skin that is yellow in color, is jaundice due to a steaming of dampness and heat in the liver and gallbladder.

- Hypochondriac pricking pain in a fixed area denotes blood stasis.

- A dull aching in the hypochondrium is usually due to deficient liver-*yin*.

- Fullness over the hypochondriac region and a referring pain that occurs during coughing and spitting suggests fluid retention in the hypochondrium.
- Alternate attacks of chills and fever and feeling of fullness and discomfort in the chest and hypochondrium indicate *shaoyang* syndrome.

Stomachache. *Wan* refers to the region of the body where the stomach is situated. Disorders such as cold, heat, stagnation of food, enterositosis, stagnation of *qi*, blood stasis, and imbalance of *yin* and *yang* of the body can impair the stomach and cause a stomachache.

- A stomachache with a feeling of cold that is relieved by warmth is caused by pathogenic cold.
- A burning stomachache with halitosis and constipation is due to an overabundance of stomach-fire.
- A distending stomachache that involves the chest and hypochondrium and is accompanied by frequent belching and aggravated by anger suggests an attack of the stomach by the hyperactive liver-*qi*.
- Epigastric distending pain accompanied by a disgust at smell of food is due to food stagnation in the gastrointestinal tract.
- A localized pricking pain in epigastric region indicates blood stasis.
- A dull aching in the stomach with desire for warmth and pressure denotes insufficient stomach-*yang*.
- A burning pain in the stomach that accompanies hunger and red tongue with little fur is indicative of deficient stomach-*yin*.

Abdominal Pain. The abdominal cavity is divided into two parts: upper abdomen and lower abdomen.

The upper abdomen is situated above the umbilicus and contains the liver, gallbladder, spleen, and stomach. Pain in the upper abdomen is often related to these organs.

The lower abdomen is located below the umbilicus and contains the kidneys, bladder, large and small intestines, and the uterus. Pain in the lower abdomen is often related to the above-mentioned organs.

Lumbago. Since the loins are referred to as the residence of the kidneys, lumbago is usually related to kidney diseases.

- A lingering pain and weakness in the loins is lumbago due to kidney-deficiency.

- Pain and a feeling of cold and heaviness in the waist that is aggravated on a cloudy and rainy day pertain to bi-syndrome due to invasion of cold-dampness.
- Lumbago radiating to the lower limbs is frequently due to blockages of channels.

Pain of Extremities. Arthritis is a bi-syndrome that often results from an attack of the meridians by pathogenic wind, cold and dampness, or heat-transformation from persistent stagnation of the three pathogens.

- A wandering pain in the joints is known as migratory arthritis. It is predominantly due to pathogenic wind and results in acute and intolerable pain.
- A heavy feeling of an affected area and localized pain is called fixed arthritis. Pathogenic dampness causes it.
- Arthritis that is accompanied by redness, swelling, heat, and joint pains and is accompanied by fever and thirst is called heat-type arthritis. Dampness transformed to heat causes it.

Distending Pain. Pain with distension is indicative of *qi* stagnation. Intermittent and migrating distending pain of the chest, hypochondrium, epigastrium, and abdomen is usually due to the stagnation of *qi* that is closely related to the function of the liver to govern normal flow of *qi*. Distending headache accompanied by slight aversion to cold, high fever, thirst, and dark urine is caused by upward attack of wind-heat; and distending pain of the eyes mostly indicates hyperactivity of liver-*yang*.

Pricking Pain. Pricking pain that is like the stabbing of a thorn is a clinical characteristic of blood stasis, often caused by trauma or stagnation of *qi* leading to the accumulation of blood in localized regions.

- A pricking headache suggests blood stasis in the head due mostly to trauma.
- A stabbing pain in the chest usually indicates an obstruction of the heart-blood.
- A twinge in the hypochondrium indicates a long depression of liver-*qi* and obstruction of blood circulation.
- A prickle sensation in the lower abdomen is indicative of blood stasis in the lower-*jiao* and is often associated with disorders of menses in women.

Colicky Pain. Colicky pain is a sudden violent pain. Generally it is caused by a sudden blockage of *qi* due to substantial pathogens or coagulation by pathogenic cold.

- Colicky pain in the pericardial area is called real cardiac pain due to an obstruction of the heart channels.
- Abdominal colicky pains with a visible mass and even vomiting of roundworms results from an upward disturbance of ascaris.
- Colicky pain in the lower abdomen accompanied by urine with sand or a sudden stop of urination indicates stranguria due to urinary stone.

Burning Pain. The flow of pathogenic fire in collaterals or hyperactivity of fire due to *yin* deficiency causes pain accompanied by a burning sensation.

- Burning pain in the stomach indicates excessiveness of stomach-fire, often accompanied by hyperorexia, halitosis and constipation.
- Burning pain in the hypochondrium, marked by irritability and acid regurgitation, suggests stagnation of the liver-fire.
- Painful and dripping urination with burning sensation is indicative of stranguria.

Cold Pain.

- Pain with cold sensation results from the body's inability to be warmed due to weakness of *yang-qi*, an inner overabundance of *yin*-cold, and an attack of meridians by pathogenic cold resulting in contraction of the affected vessels. Warmth alleviates this condition.
- Cold pain due to insufficient *yang* pertains to deficiency syndrome often accompanied by cold limbs and intolerance of cold; pale complexion; profuse and watery urine, and slow, deep, and weak pulse. Warming *yang* and activating *qi* treats this condition.
- Cold pain due to excess of *yin* is often accompanied by an aversion to cold, tastelessness, no thirst, and a deep and slow pulse. Warming *yang*, expelling cold, and relieving pain treats this condition.

Dull Pain. Dull and mild pain is due to deficient *qi* and blood leading to inability of organs and tissues to be warmed. It is often seen in chronic consumptive diseases that are characterized by long-lasting pain.

Radiating Pain. Radiating pain or referred pain is usually caused by blockage of meridians and results in deficient *qi* and blood. Chest pain radiating to the back or back pain to the chest accompanied by sweating, cold limbs, and faint indistinct pulse indicates chest bi-syndrome. Conversely, distending pain in the right hypochondrium radiating to the right shoulder is indicative of dampness and heat in the liver and gallbladder.

8.23 QUESTIONING ABOUT SLEEPING

The condition of sleeping is closely linked with the circulation of defensive *qi* and the fluctuations in the levels of *yin* and *yang*. In its normal condition, defensive-*qi* running into *yang* parts of the body during the day awakens people; when running into *yin* parts of the body during the night, it makes people sleep. *Yang-qi* is exuberant by day and so is *yin-qi* at night. During illness, sleeping patterns are abnormal due to a lack of coordination between *yin* and *yang*. Deficient *yin* and hyperactivity of *yang* lead to insomnia, whereas *yang* deficiency and overabundance of *yin*, to drowsiness. Consequently, abnormal sleeping may reflect the wane and wax of *yin* and *yang*.

Insomnia. Difficulty in falling asleep during the night or waking easily from sleep or even inability to sleep all night long is known as insomnia. This condition manifests as hyperactivity of *yang* due to deficient *yin*, and it leads to defensive *qi* failing to enter the *yin* parts of the body. The end result is mental derangement.

- Difficulty in falling asleep, accompanied by dysphoria, hectic fever, and lassitude in the joins and knees is indicative of breakdown of the functional coordination between the heart and kidneys. Deficient kidney-*yin* or overabundance of the heart-fire often causes this condition.

- Waking easily from sleep, accompanied by lassitude, palpitation, and feeble pulse suggests asthenia of both the heart and spleen.

- Frequent awakening, accompanied by dizziness, chest stuffiness, restlessness, and a bitter taste in the mouth indicate stagnation of the gallbladder-*qi* and disturbance of phlegm.

- Inability to sleep well at night, accompanied by epigastric distension and eructation suggests retention of undigested food in the stomach.

Drowsiness.

- Drowsiness (frequent uncontrollable sleepiness) when accompanied by dizziness and a heavy head is caused by an excess of *yin* due to *yang* deficiency or impairment of spleen-*yang* by dampness. This condition is often seen in epidemic febrile disease characterized by heat attacking the pericardium.

- Drowsiness accompanied by a lethargic state of the head and eyes results from a disturbance of the spleen due to phlegm-dampness.
- Drowsiness accompanied by poor appetite and anorexia and indicates insufficient spleen-*qi.*
- Drowsiness accompanied by extreme exhaustion and unconsciousness suggests deficient *yang* in the heart and kidneys.
- Drowsiness accompanied by delirium and skin eruptions is indicative of pathogenic heat attacking the pericardium.

8.24 QUESTIONING ABOUT DIET AND TASTE

Since the spleen and stomach perform the function of receiving and digesting food, appetite and taste are related to the functional condition of the spleen and stomach. Questioning should focus more attention on thirst: the amount of drink taken, drinking preference for hot or cold beverages, appetite, amount of food taken, and abnormal sense of taste or odor from mouth.

Thirst and Drinking. Thirst and drinking can reflect vicissitudes and the distribution of body fluid.

- Disease without thirst indicates no consumption of body fluid usually seen in cold syndrome.
- Excessive thirst with desire for cold drink suggests consumption of body fluid by excessive heat.
- Disease characterized by polydipsia, polyphagia and polyuria with emaciation is diabetes.
- Dry mouth without desire for drink is attributable to *yin* deficiency.
- Thirst but drinking only a little is due to damp-heat.
- Desire for hot drinks, but in drinking little or vomiting immediately after drinking is caused by retention of phlegm and fluid in the interior.
- Dry mouth with desire to gargle with water but no desire to swallow suggests accumulation of blood stasis.

Appetite and Amount of Food.

- Poor appetite with tastelessness shows deficient spleen *qi* and stomach-*qi.*

- Loss of appetite with epigastric distention, lassitude and heaviness in the head and limbs indicates impairment of the spleen by pathogenic dampness.
- Anorexia with disgust for greasy food, jaundice, and hypochondriac pain is due to dampness-heat of the liver and gallbladder.
- Disgust at smell of food accompanied by eructation and abdominal distension suggests indigestion.
- Hyperorexia with halitosis and constipation indicates excessiveness of the stomach-fire.
- Anorexia with hunger sensation and gastric discomfort is indicative of deficient stomach-*yin*.
- Preference for eating strange things is often seen in malnutrition due to parasitic infestation in children.
- Improvement of appetite in a course of disease indicates gradual recovery of stomach-*qi* and a favorable prognosis.

Taste.
- Tastelessness in the mouth is caused by deficient spleen-*qi* and stomach-*qi*.
- Sweet taste with stickiness in the mouth suggests accumulation of dampness-heat in the spleen and stomach.
- Sour taste in the mouth indicates the depressed heat in the liver and stomach.
- Acid regurgitation with foul breath signifies indigestion.
- Bitter taste in the mouth is usually indicative of overabundance of the gallbladder-fire.

8.25 Questioning about Defecation and Urination

Questioning is conducted mainly on frequency, amount, and character of feces and urine and feeling during defecation and urination.
- Constipation accompanied by high fever and abdominal distending pain pertains to excess-heat syndrome.
- *Yin* deficiency and habitual constipation in the elderly cause dry stool accompanied by red tongue with a little fur, mostly by deficient *qi*.
- Poor appetite accompanied by abdominal distension and diarrhea is attributed to insufficient spleen.
- Morning diarrhea suggests abdominal pain, mostly to insufficient kidney-*yang*.
- Diarrhea with offensive odor and abdominal pain relieved after diarrhea is due to dyspepsia.

- Frequent passage of bloody stool with pus and tenesmus indicates dysentery.
- Increased amount of urine with intolerance of cold and preference for warmth pertains to deficiency-cold syndrome.
- Urine accompanied by polydipsia, polyphagia and emaciation is known as diabetes.
- Oliguria with scanty dark urine pertains to heat-syndrome.
- Dysuria with a puffy body is a condition called edema.
- Frequent urination is often due to retention of dampness in the lower-*jiao* or a lack of consolidated kidney-*qi*.
- Urine retention leads to a condition known as anuria often caused by dampness-heat, blood stasis, or urinary stone.
- Difficult and painful urination is called straiguria.
- Frequent and dripping urination is seen in the elderly.

8.26 QUESTIONING ABOUT MENSTRUATION AND LEUKORRHEA

Questioning is conducted mainly on frequency, amount, and character of menses and feeling during menstruation.

- Menstruation occurring earlier for more than one week at every cycle is known as preceded menstrual cycle and is often due to pathogenic heat or *qi*-deficiency.
- Menstruation occurring later for more than one week at every cycle is known as delayed menstrual cycle and is often brought about by coagulation of pathogenic cold, blood stasis, deficient *yin*, or inadequate blood.
- Irregular menstruation or menstruation occurring at irregular intervals usually results from stagnation of liver-*qi* or injury of both the spleen and the kidneys.
- Scanty menstruation is due mostly to blood-deficiency, coagulation of cold, or phlegm-dampness.
- Menorrhagia is chiefly due to deficient *qi*, blood-heat, or blood stasis.
- Light red and thin discharge indicates blood-deficiency.
- Deep red and viscous menses suggests blood heat.
- Dark purplish menstrual flow with blood clots is caused by blood stasis due to coagulation of cold.

Leukorrhea. Under normal conditions discharge, if any, from the vagina is an odorless and milky white liquid. However, excessive or continuous vaginal discharge is said to be abnormal.

- Profuse or persistent vaginal discharge with whitish and clear tinge is called leukorrhea and is seepage of dampness due to spleen-asthenia.

- Yellowish, viscid and foul discharge from the vagina is called yellowish leukorrhagia and is attributed to the downward flow of damp-heat.

- Leukorrhagia with blood and pus is called reddish leukorrhagia is due primarily to stagnated heat of the liver channel.

8.27 Questioning about the Condition of a Child

Besides routine questioning, questions concerning general status before and after the birth, the history of vaccination, and the child's history of infectious diseases are also necessary. In the case of neonatal disorders, a pregnant woman should be questioned as to her nutritive state and delivery condition; in the case of infant diseases, ask about feeding habits and growth condition.

- The child who has already been vaccinated or who has acquired a long-term immunity to a disease after having had it previously will not contract it a second time.

- A child not exposed to vaccine or who has already experienced a long-term immunity is liable to contract the disease if he or she is exposed to it recently.

- Infants are liable to be frightened since their minds are not fully developed.

- They are susceptible to indigestion because of weakness of the spleen and stomach.

- They are prone to be affected by seasonal pathogens due to inability to adapt to changes in the weather.

8.28 Taking the Pulse

Taking one's pulse is a diagnostic procedure by which a doctor examines the pulse condition to detect the condition of an illness and gathers clinical data through palpating the pulsation of the radial arteries with his or her fingertips.

Three Portions and Nine Pulse-Takings. This term has two meanings in TCM.

1. A diagnostic method of general pulse-feelings. The three parts of the body to be palpated are the head, the hand, and the foot, each of which, in turn, is subdivided into three portions: upper, middle, and lower. In other words there are altogether nine parts of the body to be palpated for diagnostic purposes.

The concrete portions are in the head portion:

- The upper (heaven) temporal artery at point *taiyang* (Extra2) to detect the temporal *qi* *The middle (human) auricular artery at point *ermen* (SJ2) to detect the *qi* of eye and ear.

- The lower (earth) buccal artery at point *ju liao* (S3) to detect the *qi* of mouth and teeth.

- Likewise, similar portions exist in the hand:

- The upper (heaven) radial artery of lung meridian at *cunkou* to detect the lung *qi.*

- The middle (human) ulnar artery of heart meridian at point *shenmen* (H7) to detect heart-*qi.*

- The lower (earth) artery of large intestine meridians at point *hegu* (L14) to detect the pectoral-*qi.*

Finally, in the foot portion, one would palpate:

- The upper (heaven) artery of liver meridian at point *wuli* (Liv 10) or *taichong* (Liv 3) to detect liver-*qi.*

- The middle (human) artery of spleen meridian at point *jinien* (S11) or *chongyang* (S42) to detect the *qi* of the spleen and stomach.

- The lower (earth) artery of kidney meridian at point *taixi* (K3) to detect the kidney *qi.*

2. Pulse-taking on *cunkou* is a general term for the three pulse locations on the wrist over the radial artery. Specifically, these three points are *cun*, *guan* and *chi*, and each location is palpated with light, moderate and heavy pressure respectively to get nine aspects of the pulse condition.

Cun, Guan,* and *Chi. *Cun*, *guan*, and *chi* (inch, bar, and cubit) are the three places on the wrist over the radial artery where the pulse is felt. Concretely, *guan* is located over the prominent head of the radius at the wrist; *cun* is adjacent to it on the distal side, while *chi* is on the proximal side.

Correspondence between *Cun, Guan,* and *Chi* and Viscera.
The three pulses of *cun*, *guan*, and *chi* indicate the states of the five *zang* organs and six *fu* organs. The three pulses of the left hand can reflect conditions of the heart, (the pericardium), the liver (the gallbladder and diaphragm), the kidneys (especially kidney-*yin*), and the lower abdomen respectively. Those of the right hand indicate conditions of the lungs (thorax), the spleen (the stomach), the kidneys (especially kidney-*yang*), and the lower abdomen.

Method of Feeling the Pulse.

1. Time. The best time for pulse-feeling is the early morning because the patient is then less affected by food intake and other activities and qi and blood in meridians are less disturbed, thus making it easy to recognize a patient's real pulse. However, in other times, pulse can also be felt. Generally speaking, pulse-feeling requires a quiet environment and a patient in a calm mood with stable qi and blood in order for an accurate diagnosis to be made.

2. Position of the body. The patient is required to sit or lie flat on the back with the arm extending, the palm facing upward and the forearm being on nearly the same level as the heart in order to keep *qi* and blood flowing freely. Meanwhile, the cloth pillow should be placed under the patient's wrist for convenience of pulse-feeling.

3. Arrangement of the fingers. The physician should put his or her index, middle, and ring fingers on the patient's three pulse portions of *cun*, *guan*, and *chi* for adults. The tip of the middle finger is first put over *guan* region, that of the index finger over the *cun* region, and that of the ring finger over the *chi* region. The distances among the three fingers should be adjusted according to the patient's height. Use just one finger (index finger or thumb) to feel the pulse for children over three years of age. Additionally, observation of the superficial venules of their index fingers is made instead of pulse-feeling for infants under three years.

4. Manipulations. Pulse-taking is made by pressing the arteries with the palm surfaces of the three fingers, which are slightly bent like bows so that the tips of the three fingers are at the same level. Recognition of pulse condition is made usually through applying three grades of finger forces on the three pulse regions. First, the finger force is exerted lightly, a procedure named touching, then moderate force is applied (called searching), and finally heavier pressure is exerted, i.e., general pressing.

   In order to recognize the pulse condition of one particular portion, one of the three fingers can be used alone to feel the pulse. This is known as individual pressing. Clinically, general pressing is often applied in combination with individual pressing.

5. Duration of pulse-taking. Three to five minutes are enough for each feeling, and the minimum time for pulse-feeling should be no less than one minute.

Normal Pulse. Normal pulse refers to the pulse condition of a healthy person, characterized by its stomach-*qi*, vitality, and root.

- When the pulse is moderate, unhurried, calm, and regular, it is said to have stomach-*qi*.
- Soft, even and forceful pulse indicates the pressure and interior syndrome.
- Deep and forceful pulse indicates an interior-excess syndrome in which the pathogens accumulate in the interior and *qi* and blood are stagnated.
- Deep and forceless pulse suggests an interior-deficiency syndrome in which weakness of *zang-fu* organs and insufficient *qi* and blood lead to inability of channel-*qi* to be activated.

Hidden Pulse. Hidden pulse is one felt only on pressing the bone hard is located even deeper than deep pulse, and is seen in cases of syncope. Severe pains result from accumulation of pathogens in the interior of the body, which bring about the obstructions of *qi* and blood. If a pulse cannot be felt on *cunkou* of both the left and right sides nor on the points *taixi* and *fuyang*, the case is critical.

Firm Pulse. Firm pulse is forceful, large, taut, and long. It is felt only by pressing hard and is usually seen in obstinate diseases with accumulation of *yin* cold, such as abdominal mass and hernia. The firm pulse that results from the sinking of *yang-qi* and coagulation of *yin* cold inside the body reflects solidity and excessiveness of pathogens belonging to excess syndrome.

Detection of stomach-*qi*, vitality, and root in pulse condition has certain clinical significance in the improvement or deterioration and favorable or unfavorable prognosis of a disease. Meanwhile, with changes in the body's internal and environmental factors, normal pulse often undergoes physiological changes.

The following pulses are physiological variations of a firm and normal pulse rather than abnormal pulses (as listed in the next section).

- Because of seasonal variations, the pulse in spring is somewhat taut; in summer somewhat full; in autumn somewhat floating; and in winter somewhat deep.
- Strenuous exercise, emotional excitement, eating and drinking often cause the pulse to speed up.
- An anatomic anomaly of the radial artery makes the pulse beat run from the *chi* area laterally and obliquely to *hukou* (near point *hegu*) on the back of the hand is called slantly-located radial pulse.

- Radial pulse palpable at the dorsum of the wrist in an anomaly of the radial artery is named ectopic radial pulse.

Abnormal Pulse. The pulse condition reflecting various pathological changes of a diseased body is known as an abnormal pulse. Following are several abnormal pulse conditions.

Floating Pulse. Floating pulse is one that can be felt only by light touch and that grows faint on pressing hard, usually indicating exterior syndrome and deficiency syndrome as well. It is often seen in the common cold and in the early stage of an acute febrile disease, in which the defensive *qi* resists the pathogens on the body surface and, thus, channel-*qi* becomes more superficial. In a weak patient with a prolonged illness, the floating pulse suggests the consumption of essence-*qi*. This condition promotes *yin*'s failure to keep *yang* well or to release sufficient *yang* to the exterior.

Hollow Pulse. A pulse that feels floating, large and hollow is mainly seen in cases marked by severe hemorrhage or exhaustion of body fluid due to profuse sweating. This condition results in outward floating of *yang-qi* that loses its foundation due to abrupt consumption of blood or *yin*-fluid.

Scattered Pulse. Scattered pulse is a pulse condition with scattered and disordered beats and without root. It can be felt only by light touch and becomes impalpable by heavy pressure, as seen in critical cases, and indicates depletion of primordial *qi* and exhaustion of *qi* of *zang-fu* organs.

Deep Pulse. Deep pulse is a pulse condition in which the beats are located deep and are hard to feel by light touch.

- Deep pulse becomes distinct by hard pressure indicating interior-excess syndrome.
- Pathogens accumulate in the interior and *qi* and blood stagnate.
- Deep and forceless pulse suggests an interior-deficiency syndrome, in which weakness of the *zang-fu* organs and insufficient *qi* and blood lead to an inability of channel-*qi* to be activated.

Slow Pulse. Slow pulse is one with less than four beats to a normal cycle of respiration (less than sixty beats per minute), indicating cold syndrome. Sometimes slow pulse also suggests aggregation of pathogenic heat leading to the stagnancy of *qi*-blood, as seen in excess-heat syndrome of *yangming fu* organs.

- Slow and forceful pulse indicates excess syndrome due to accumulation of cold causing the stagnation of *qi*.

- Slow and feeble pulse suggests insufficient *yin-qi* and deficiency-cold syndrome.
- Slow but vigorous pulse palpated in a well-trained athlete is considered normal.

Moderate Pulse. Moderate pulse is one characterized by four beats to one cycle of respiration, with even rhythm and moderate tension and seen in damp syndrome. Under this condition, dampness obstructs *qi*-blood in circulation or promotes weakness of the spleen and stomach, which fail to promote the normal flow of *qi*-blood. The pulse of a patient beating gently and moderately indicates the recovery of the patient's vital *qi*.

Rapid Pulse. Rapid pulse is one with five to six beats to a normal cycle of respiration (from 91-120 beats per minute), generally indicating heat syndrome and swift flow of *qi* and blood due to pathogenic heat.

- Rapid and strong pulse indicates excess-heat syndrome as a result of a fierce struggle between heat pathogens and the undiminished body resistance.
- Rapid and feeble pulse indicates deficiency-heat syndrome and results from *yin* deficiency due to protracted illness.
- Rapid, large, forceless, and hollow pulse when felt with pressure suggests a disease marked by outward floating of deficient *yang*.

Swift Pulse. A swift pulse is hasty and quick, with over seven beats to a normal cycle of respiration (more than 121 beats per minute). A swift pulse indicates exhaustion of *yin* or prostration of primordial *qi* due to overabundance of *yang* and is often seen in the climax of a febrile disease and a consumptive disease with exhausted *yin* failing to keep *yang*. In short, swift pulse is indicative of an extremely critical condition.

- Swift and hard pulse suggests extreme consumption of *yin* due to hyperactivity of *yang* beyond control.
- Swift and feeble pulse indicates immediate prostration of vital *qi*.

Feeble Pulse. Feeble pulse is a general term for all forceless pulses that feel soft, weak, and hollow, when pressing either lightly or heavily on *cun*, *guan*, and *chi*. This condition indicates deficiency syndrome, often seen in:

- Deficient *qi* and blood, especially insufficient *qi* that is unable to promote blood circulation.
- Weakness of *zang-fu* organs.

Replete Pulse. Replete pulse, a general term for all vigorous pulses, feels vigorous and forceful at *cun*, *guan*, and *chi* with both light and hard pressure. This condition indicates excess syndrome, in which overabundant pathogens struggle against the strong vital *qi* and give rise to stagnation of *qi* and blood and excessive repletion of the channels.

Slippery Pulse. Slippery pulse comes and goes smoothly. It feels slick to the finger like beads rolling on a plate and indicates excess-heat syndrome, phlegm retention, and dyspepsia. Slippery and moderate pulse occurring in a healthy person suggests plentitude and free flow of nutritive *qi* and defensive-*qi*. In addition, it is also seen in a pregnant woman and shows the adequacy and harmony of *qi* and blood.

Hesitant Pulse. A hesitant pulse does not come and go smoothly. It is like scraping bamboo with a knife. Its condition is just the opposite of slippery pulse.

- Hesitant and forceless pulse indicates deficient essence and blood, which leads to the emptiness of vessels and obstruction of blood flow.

- Hesitant and forceful pulse is indicative of stagnancy of *qi* and blood stasis or persistent retention of phlegm or food, which hinders *qi*-blood from free circulation.

Thready Pulse. Thready pulse, also called small pulse, is as thin as a silk thread and feeble, yet easily perceptible. It usually indicates one of two syndromes: deficient *qi* and blood or chronic deficiency. Essentially, an inadequate blood supply fails to adequately replenish the vessels. Additionally, weak *qi* fails to impel blood to flow. Thready pulse may also be attributed to dampness disease in which the pathogenic dampness constricts the vessels and impedes the channel *qi*.

- Thready and feeble pulse is often seen in blood-deficiency syndrome.

- Thready and rapid pulse is found in *yin*-deficiency syndrome.

- If a thready and rapid pulse appears in cases with seasonal febrile disease accompanied by coma and delirium, it indicates invasion of *ying* (nutrient) system and *xue* (blood) system or an attack of the pericardium by pathogenic heat.

Soft Pulse. A soft pulse feels floating, thready and forceless by light touch, but faint upon pressing heavily. It indicates both deficiency syndrome and dampness syndrome. In the deficiency syndrome, deficient nutritive *qi* and blood fail to replenish the vessels and prevent *qi* from flowing outward. In dampness syndrome, soft pulse originates from insufficient *qi*-blood and invasion of exogenous dampness resulting in outward dispersing of *yang-qi*.

Indistinct Pulse. A pulse with extremely thready and soft beats, only palpable faintly, is called an indistinct pulse. It indicates the depletion of *qi*, sudden prostration of *yang*, and other severe deficiency syndromes.

- When an indistinct pulse occurs in a protracted disease, it is indicative of exhaustion of vital-*qi* often seen in patients with decline of kidney-*yang* and heart-*yang*.
- When an indistinct pulse appears in a recent attack of disease, it indicates abrupt collapse of *yang-qi*.

Weak Pulse. A weak pulse is extremely soft, deep and thready and is seen in patients experiencing deficient *qi* and blood.

- Weak pulse appearing in a prolonged disease indicates a favorable prognosis due to correspondence of a pulse to a syndrome.
- Weak pulse in a new disease is due to excessive pathogens and indicates that the disease will have an unfavorable prognosis due to the pulse's failure to correspond to the syndrome.

Full Pulse. Full pulse is forceful like waves surging, coming vigorously and going gently with a large volume. It usually indicates a preponderance of pathogenic heat in the *qi* system. Because excessive of heat inside the body promotes accumulation of *qi* and blood and dilation of the vessels, the pulse becomes large, floating and forceful and the heat comes vigorously and goes gently. If full pulse appears in a protracted disease with consumption of *qi*, blood loss, or protracted diarrhea, it suggests a crisis due to violence of pathogens and deficient vital *qi*.

Large Pulse. A pulse with a wave that lifts the fingertip to a great height but does not tend to surge quite as high as a full pulse is called large pulse.

- Large and forceful pulse suggests excess syndrome of pathogenic heat.
- Large and weak pulse indicates deficiency syndrome marked by vital *qi*'s failure to be kept inside the body.

Taut Pulse. A taut pulse feels straight and long, hard like the string of a musical instrument. It is usually seen in cases of the liver and gallbladder troubles, various pain syndromes, and retention of phlegm and fluid.

- When the liver and gallbladder are troubled, the function may be impaired, losing the moderation of liver-*qi*, thereby forming the taut pulse.
- When pains and phlegm exist, taut pulse is the sign of the stagnation of *qi*.

- Taut pulse is also seen in malaria, consumptive disease or internal injury; insufficient *qi* of middle-*jiao*, and hyperactive liver-*qi*'s attack on the spleen.
- If a pulse feels taut, thready and rapid like the edge of a knife, the disease will be difficult to treat because of complete loss of stomach-*qi*.
- A soft, moderate, and taut pulse appearing in a healthy person in spring is considered normal.

Tense Pulse. A tense pulse is strained and forceful, like a stretched twisted cord. It usually indicates cold syndrome. Pathogenic cold in the exterior often manifests as a floating and tense pulse. Pathogenic cold in the interior by deep and tense pulse. A tense pulse also appears in cases of acute pain or retention of undigested food.

Tympanic Pulse. An extremely taut and hollow pulse that feels like touching the surface of a drum is called a tympanic pulse. It is often seen in patients with depletion of blood or spermatorrhea, abortion, metrorrhagia, or metrostaxis, which all lead to outward floating of *qi* resulting from exhaustion of essence and blood.

Intermittent Pulse. A slow and weak pulse pausing at regular intervals is called intermittent pulse and is often seen in cases of visceral dysfunction, especially weakness of the heart-*qi*. This condition gives rise to the inability of the channel-*qi* to continue regularly and appears in wind syndrome, pain syndrome, persistent and violent emotions, and trauma due to suspension of channel-*qi* (which should not be considered as severe conditions).

Running Pulse. A swift pulse with irregular intermittence is called a running pulse. Running and forceful pulse usually suggests heat-syndrome due to an overabundance of *yang*. Stagnancy of *qi* and blood, retention of phlegm, or indigestion causes this condition. Attention should be paid to the running, thready, and weak pulse, which is indicative of prostratin syndrome.

Knotted Pulse. A slow and uneven pulse pausing at irregular intervals is called a knotted pulse. It indicates *qi* stagnation due to excess *yin*, such as cold-phlegm syndrome, blood stasis, and abdominal mass. The obstruction or aggregation of *qi* and blood, coagulation of phlegm by cold, and blockage of channel-*qi* cause knotted pulse

Long and Short Pulse. Long pulse is characterized by a prolonged stroke.

- Long and gentle pulse reflecting sufficient *qi* of middle-*jiao* and free flow of *qi* and blood is considered normal.

- Long and taut pulse indicates an excess syndrome, such as hyperactivity of the liver *yang* or accumulation of pathogenic heat in the interior due to overabundance of *yang*.

- pulse with short extent, only palpable at the *guan* site but indistinct at *cun* and *chi* is called short pulse, the condition of which is just opposite to a long pulse.

- Short and forceful pulse formed by the failure of obstructed channel-*qi* to extend normally indicates stagnation of *qi*, blood stasis and retention of phlegm or dyspepsia.

- Short and weak pulse results from an inability of weak *qi* to promote blood flowing with vigor suggesting consumption and deficient *qi*.

Tremulous Pulse. A pulse that feels short, slippery, quick, and forceful (like a bouncing pea) is called a tremulous pulse and is seen in cases of terror and pain syndrome and results from a lack of coordination between *yin* and *yang* and disorder of both *qi* and blood.

Coexisting Pulse. A pulse composed of two or more pulse conditions existing simultaneously is called a coexisting pulse. Generally speaking, a coexisting pulse indicates a collection of diseases that each single pulse indicates. For example, floating and tense pulse indicates exterior cold syndrome and deep, thready, and rapid pulse suggests interior heavy syndrome of the deficiency type.

Deteriorated Pulse. A pulse without stomach-*qi*, vitality, and root is known as deteriorated pulse indicative of the depletion of vital *qi* of *zang-fu* organs and exhaustion of stomach-*qi*. It is usually seen during a patient's dying stage. Therefore, it is also known as moribund pulse. Since its condition is peculiar and quite different from ordinary pulse condition, it is also named strange pulse.

Seven Moribund Pulses. Seven moribund pulses refer to the pulse conditions seen in critical cases, i.e., bubble-rising pulse, fish-swimming pulse, shrimp-darting pulse, roof-leaking pulse, bird-pecking pulse, rope-untying pulse, and knocking-stone pulse. These are described below.

Ten Strange Pulses. Wei Yilin, a distinguished physician of the Yuan dynasty, described ten moribund pulses. They include the seven moribund pulses indicated above and the knife-edge, pea-rolling, and confused running pulses.

Bubble-rising Pulse. Bubble-rising pulse refers to a floating pulse beating like bubbles rising to the surface of boiling water. It indicates exhaustion of *yin*-fluid due to extreme overabundance of heat of the three *yang* channels.

Fish-swimming Pulse. Fish-swimming pulse is hardly perceptible (like a swimming fish). It is indicative of outward depletion of *yang* due to extreme overabundance of cold of the three *yin* channels.

Shrimp-darting Pulse. Shrimp-darting pulse refers to a nearly imperceptible pulse with occasional darting beats that resemble a shrimp darting in water. It indicates outward floating of solitary *yang* and exhaustion of *qi* of the large intestine.

Roof-leaking Pulse. Roof-leaking pulse refers to a quite slow and arrhythmic pulse like the drops of rain that leak through the roof. It indicates the exhaustion of stomach-*qi*.

Bird-pecking Pulse. Bird-pecking pulse beats with rapid, irregular rhythms like a bird pecking food. It indicates exhaustion of spleen-*qi*.

Rope-untying Pulse. Rope-untying pulse is an irregular and rhythmless pulse resembling the untying of a knotted rope. It indicates depletion of both kidney-*qi* and *qi* of *mingmen*.

Knocking-stone Pulse. Knocking-stone pulse is deep and solid yet forceless and feels like flicking a stone with the fingertips. It indicates exhaustion of kidney-*qi*.

Prognosis according to the Relationship between Pulse and Symptoms. The pulse condition corresponding to the symptoms indicates a favorable prognosis while that which does not correspond to the symptoms, an unfavorable prognosis. As examples:

- Full, rapid, and replete pulse occurring in an excess syndrome is a favorable case showing that the strong body resistance preponderates over the pathogens.

- Small, indistinct and weak pulse in an excess syndrome is a deteriorating case with pathogens overpowering the body's resistance.

- Floating, full, rapid, and replete pulse occurring in a newly-contracted or acute disease indicates that the pulse corresponds to the symptoms and the strong vital *qi* can defeat the pathogens.

- Deep, small, indistinct, and weak pulse occurring in a recently-developed or acute disease suggests that the pulse does not correspond to the symptoms and the vital *qi* has declined.

- Deep, indistinct, thready, and weak pulse appearing in a prolonged disease indicates that the pulse corresponds to the symptoms, and the vital *qi* recovers with retreat of the pathogens.

- Full, rapid, and replete pulse in a protracted disease indicates that the pulse does not correspond to the symptoms, and the vital *qi* declines without retreat of the pathogens.

8.29 PALPATION OF THE BODY

Palpation of the body is a diagnostic procedure by which a doctor can palpate the patient's skin, limbs, chest, abdomen, and other affected regions of the body to detect local abnormal changes and thereby determine the location and nature of the disease.

Palpation of the Skin.

- Fever that rises at the first palpation but lowers after a long press indicates heat syndrome of the skin.
- Low fever that increases as the length of the palpation extends suggests heat syndrome of the interior.
- Swelling skin that caves in and fails to recover after it is pressed indicates edema.
- Swelling skin that leaves an impression when pressed but that disappears at once after the hand has been withdrawn is indicative of edema due to *qi* stagnation.

Palpation of the Extremities. The nature of a disorder can also be detected by palpating or feeling the extremities. For instance:

- Cold of both hands and feet indicates excess of *yin* due to *yang* deficiency pertaining to cold syndrome.
- Cold limbs may also be caused by failure of *yang-qi* to reach the limbs due to accumulation of interior heat.
- Fever in both hands and feet is indicative of either over-abundance of *yang* or *yin* deficiency, pertaining to heat syndrome.

By palpating the extremities a doctor is also able to differentiate diseases due to exogenous pathogens from those due to internal injury. As examples:

- Fever in dorsal surface of the hands and feet is due to affection by exogenous pathogens.
- in palms and soles that is higher than the fever in the forehead suggests internal injury. Moreover, by palpating the temperature of limbs a doctor can also detect the presence or depletion of *yang-qi* and predict prognosis of disorders due to *yang* deficiency.

- A *yang* deficiency syndrome with warm limbs is curable because of presence of *yang-qi*.
- A *yang* deficiency syndrome with cold limbs often has an unfavorable prognosis.

Palpation of *Xuli*. The *xuli* area (over the apex of the heart) is the site where pectoral-*qi* converges and stomach-*qi* accumulates. Under normal conditions, the *xuli* pulse is vigorous but not tense, moderate but not rapid. It indicates accumulation of the pectoral-*qi* in the chest.

- Small and weak *xuli* pulse is due to internal insufficient pectoral-*qi*.
- Excessively strong *xuli* pulse suggests the release of pectoral-*qi*.
- Retained fluid blocking the pericardium may also cause an indistinct pulse.

Palpation of Epigastrium. By palpating the epigastrium for its hardness and tenderness upon pressure, a doctor differentiates the fullness syndrome from syndromes due to the accumulation of pathogens in the chest. For example, a feeling of epigastric pain, distension, and rigidity upon the application of pressure is referred to as a syndrome of accumulation of pathogens in chest, while softness and no pain sensation upon applying pressure is described as a syndrome of fullness.

Palpation of Abdomen.

- Abdominal distension with a tympanic note on percussion but with normal urination indicates *qi*-distention.
- Abdominal distension like that of a water bag upon pressure with dysuria suggests ascites.
- Hard and immovable mass found in the abdomen with fixed pain is due to the disease of the blood system due to blood stasis.
- A mass in the abdomen that appears or disappears alternatively and that is movable but without fixed pain pertains to disease of the *qi* system due to stagnation of *qi*.

In addition, by palpating the abdomen, a doctor can differentiate abdominal pain of a deficiency type from that of an excess type and detect acute appendicitis, malnutrition due to parasitic infestation and dry stool in the large intestine.

Palpation of Acupoints. Acupoints are the small pools of the circulating *qi*-blood of meridians in the skin and the sites where the *qi* of the *zang-fu* organs passes. Palpating of acupoints provides doctors with information as to changes and responses in the internal organs and thereby facilitates the diagnosis of diseases of internal organs.

Tenderness and sensitive reactions upon palpating the corresponding acupoint chiefly indicate nodes in the corresponding acupoint and abnormal responses.

CHAPTER 9

Differential Diagnosis

9.1 *BAGANG BIANZHENG* (DIAGNOSIS IN ACCORDANCE WITH THE EIGHT PRINCIPAL SYNDROMES)

To recap: The eight principal syndromes are: exterior or interior, cold or heat and deficient or excessive, *yin* or *yang*. *Bagang bianzheng* is a method of differential diagnosis used to determine the nature and location of pathological changes and the conflict between body resistance and pathogens in terms of the eight principal syndromes. This method focuses on a comprehensive analysis of all of the data obtained by means of inspection, auscultation and olfaction, interrogation, pulse feeling and palpation.

9.2 DIFFERENTIAL DIAGNOSIS OF INTERIOR OR EXTERIOR SYNDROME

A method of differential diagnosis used to determine the action of pathological changes and the development tendency of a disease.

Exterior Syndrome. Exterior syndrome is caused by an attack of the superficies by six exogenous pathogens through the skin, hair, mouth, and nose. It is sudden in onset, superficial and mild in nature, and short in duration without affecting the function of *zang-fu* organs in most cases.

Interior Syndrome. Interior syndrome is characterized by pathological changes of the internal organs caused by pathogens. Interior syndrome is produced by:

- Exogenous pathogens that either enter the interior from the superficies or directly invade the *zang-fu* organs.
- Other factors that affect the functions of *zang-fu* organs, such as emotional upset, improper diet, or overstrain.

Invasion from the Exterior to the Interior. Invasion from the exterior to the interior includes the invasion of pathogens from the superficial part of the body to the deep parts, or the replacement of exterior syndrome by interior one. For example, a patient with exterior syndrome exhibits symptoms such as fever, a chilly sensation, thin fur of the tongue, and floating pulse. However, sometimes the chilly sensation is replaced by aversion to heat and other symptoms—such as thirst, scanty dark urine, redness of the tongue with yellowish fur, and rapid pulse. In this case, the disease has manifested itself by interior heat syndrome due to invasion of pathogenic agents from the superficial part of the body to the deep.

Invasion from the Interior to the Skin. Invasion from the interior to the skin refers to the condition in which the pathogenic agent is brought out from the interior to the skin. The transmission of pathogens from the interior to the skin is indicative of convalescence of a disease in which the pathogens have been in expelled and condition of the illness has abated.

For example, in the case of an interior syndrome due to interior heat, the patient exhibits restlessness, shortness of breath, cough, and chest stuffiness. Later, fever and sweat and the interior syndrome subside. This change indicates that the pathogenic agent has been brought out. It usually results from proper and prompt treatment and appropriate nursing, which help to build up body resistance.

Coexistence of Exterior Syndrome and Interior Syndrome. A coexistence of exterior and interior syndromes refers to simultaneous appearance of both exterior syndrome and interior syndrome in a patient. It may result from the following conditions:

- Both exterior syndrome and interior syndrome appear in the initial stage of an illness For example, in late summer or early autumn an invasion by external pathogenic cold and internal pathogenic damp may cause exterior and interior syndrome symptoms to appear. In this case, exterior symptoms include fever, chilly sensation, headache and general aching, and interior symptoms include epigastric stuffiness, anorexia, diarrhea, and thick, whitish tongue fur.

- The illness involves the exterior first and then affects the interior.

- Interior syndrome is complicated by an attack of exogenous pathogens or improper diet complicates initial invasion by exopathogens.

9.3 DIFFERENTIAL DIAGNOSIS OF COLD AND HEAT SYNDROMES

Differential diagnosis of cold and heat syndromes is a method of differentiating the nature of a disease. It is identical with the differentiation of excess and deficient *yin* and *yang*, because cold and heat are the manifestations of excess and deficient *yin* and *yang* in the body.

Cold Syndrome. Invasion of the pathogenic cold or hypofunction of the body due to insufficient *yang* and excess *yin* causes cold syndrome. This condition is marked by aversion to cold or preference for warmth, no thirst, pale complexion, huddling up with cold, copious clear urine, loose stools, pale tongue with whitish fur, and tense or slow pulse.

Heat Syndrome. Invasion of pathogenic heat or hyperactivity of the body due to deficient *yin* and excess *yang* causes heat syndrome. It is marked by fever; aversion to heat and preference for coolness; thirst with preference for cold drinks; flushed face; congested eyes; fidgets; scanty dark urine; constipation; reddened tongue with dry, brownish fur and rapid pulse.

Simultaneous Occurrence of Cold and Heat Syndromes. When cold syndrome is intertwined with heat syndrome in the same patient, it is usually classified into two types:

1. In the case of a pure interior syndrome, it is characterized by heat syndrome in the upper part with cold syndrome in the lower part of the body or vice versa.

2. In the case of simultaneous occurrence of exterior and interior syndrome, it is marked by heat syndrome in the exterior with cold syndrome in the interior or vice versa.

Transformation of Cold Syndrome and Heat Syndrome.
Transformation of cold and heat syndromes refers to a change of the nature of a disease, i.e., conversion from cold syndrome to heat syndrome or vice versa. For example, a disease can, at its onset, manifest as cold syndrome followed by heat syndrome, and the former vanishes as soon as the latter appears. This is what is known as transformation of cold syndrome into heat syndrome, as in the case of exterior cold syndrome due to exogenous pathogens. It is marked by symptoms such as fever, chilly sensation, no sweat, headache, general aching, thin whitish tongue fur, and tense floating pulse. Later, owing to further development of the pathological changes, the chilly sensation disappears but fever does not abate and an aversion to heat rather than cold occurs. Additionally, other symptoms appear one after another. These symptoms include irritability, thirst and yellowish tongue fur and indicate that the exterior cold syndrome has transformed into interior heat syndrome.

On the other hand, if a disease at its onset manifests itself by heat syndrome followed by cold syndrome, the former dies away as soon as the latter appears. This condition is called transformation of heat syndrome into cold syndrome and is exemplified by the patient with high fever who, due to delayed treatment or misdiagnosis, is overcome by pathogenic factors that prevail over vital *qi*. Suddenly this patient develops symptoms such as cold limbs, profuse cold sweat, listlessness, and faint indistinct pulse.

Heat Syndrome with Pseudo-cold Symptoms. Heat syndrome with pseudo-cold symptoms manifests as a disease of heat nature, but it exhibits some cold symptoms such as cold limbs and deep pulse. It is different from cold syndrome in that:

- The patient's body is warm in spite of cold limbs.
- He or she has an aversion to heat instead of cold.
- His or her pulse is deep, but also rapid and forceful.

The patient may also have the following symptoms: excessive thirst, preference for cold drink, dry throat, foul breath, delirium, scanty dark urine, dry stool or dysentery of heat type with rectal tenesmus, dark reddish tongue with dry yellowish fur. In this case, cold limbs and deep pulse are false appearances, while overabundant interior heat is the essence of the disease. This condition is attributable to excessive heat inside the body, which keeps *yin* superficially located.

Cold Syndrome with Pseudo-heat Symptoms. Cold syndrome with pseudo-heat symptoms manifests as a disease of cold nature, but it exhibits some heat symptoms such as fever, flushed face, thirst, and large pulse. This condition differs from heat syndrome in that the patient runs a fever, but has a desire to be covered up; he or she feels thirsty, but prefers to hot drinks and his or her pulse is large, but weak. Additional symptoms of cold nature occur, including cold limbs, clear urine, loose stool and pink tongue with whitish fur. This syndrome is caused by excessive *yin*-cold inside the body that keeps *yang* externally located.

9.4 DIFFERENTIAL DIAGNOSIS OF DEFICIENCY AND EXCESS

Differential diagnosis of deficiency and excess is a method of differential diagnosis used to determine the strength of vital *qi* of the body and the virulence of pathogenic agents.

Deficiency Syndrome. Deficiency syndrome refers to a morbid state manifested as deficient vital *qi*. It results from congenital defects and lack of proper care after birth, the latter being the main cause. For example, improper diet may lead to weakness of the physique; emotional upsets may impair *qi* and blood of *zang-fu* organs; sexual indulgence may consume the kidney *qi*; and prolonged illness may impair vital *qi*. All of these factors may result in various deficiency syndromes, which include insufficiency and impairment of *yin*, *yang*, *qi*, blood, essence of life, body fluid, and *zang-fu* organs. These conditions manifest as pale or yellowish complexion, listlessness, emaciation, fatigue and weakness, disinclination to talk, palpitation, shortness of breath, lassitude in loins and knees, spontaneous perspiration, night sweats, incontinence of stool and urine, pain relieved by pressing, pink tongue with little or no fur, and feeble or weak pulse.

Excess Syndrome. Excess syndrome refers to a morbid condition marked by exuberant pathogens. It may result from rampant pathogens struggling with vital *qi*. Its main manifestations are strong physical constitution, high fever, agitation, loud voice, abdominal distension, pain and tenderness, constipation, oliguria, rough pale tongue with thick and greasy fur, and replete and forceful pulse.

Deficiency Syndrome Complicated with Excess Syndrome. Deficiency syndrome complicated with excess syndrome refers to a simultaneous occurrence of deficiency syndrome and excess syndrome in same patient at the same time. It may be classified into three types:

1. Deficiency syndrome is dominant, complicated with excess symptoms.

2. Excess syndrome is predominant accompanied by deficiency symptoms.

3. Co-existence of excess syndrome and deficiency syndrome.

Treatment must vary and depends on the type the syndrome.

Transformation of Excess Syndrome to Deficiency Syndrome. In the case of transformation of excess syndrome to deficiency syndrome, the disease is characterized by excess syndrome in its initial stage. Due to delayed treatment or misdiagnosis, it evolves into deficiency syndrome as a result of decline of pathogens and impaired vital *qi* during the protracted course of disease. For example, if not properly treated, an excess heat syndrome consumes body fluid and *qi* during the protracted course of disease and gives rise to deficiency symptoms.

Transformation of Deficiency Syndrome to Excess Syndrome. In the case of transformation of deficiency syndrome to excess syndrome, the disease is characterized by deficiency syndrome in its early stage. Due to insufficient vital *qi*, substantial pathogens gradually accumulate inside the body and give rise to some excess symptoms.

Excess Syndrome with Pseudo-deficiency Symptoms. Excess syndrome with pseudo-deficiency symptoms is a syndrome of the excess type that is characterized by the accumulation of pathogens and accompanied by symptoms similar to deficiency syndrome.

Deficiency Syndrome with Pseudo-excess Symptoms. Deficiency syndrome with pseudo-excess symptoms is a syndrome of the deficiency type and is accompanied by symptoms similar to excess syndrome.

Exterior Syndrome of Excess Type. Exterior syndrome of the excess type is a syndrome resulting from tight closure of striae of the skin and muscles due to invasion of the skin by exogenous pathogens. This condition manifests as fever, chills, headache, general aching, stuffy nose, no sweat and tense floating pulse.

Exterior Syndrome of Deficiency Type. Exterior syndrome of the deficiency type has two connotations:

1. One connotation refers to a syndrome due to pathogens invading the body surface, complicated by disharmony between nutritive *qi* and defensive *qi* and loose muscular striae. Its clinical manifestations are fever, aversion to wind, sweating, and slow floating pulse.

2. The other connotation suggests superficial *qi*'s failure to protect the body because of deficient spleen-*qi* and lung-*qi*. As a result of *qi*-deficiency and weakened skin, the patient has spontaneous perspiration and is susceptible to exogenous pathogens.

Cold Syndrome of Deficiency Type. Cold syndrome of the deficiency type is a syndrome caused by deficient *yang-qi* and manifested by:

- Lassitude
- Pale complexion
- Aversion to cold and cold limbs
- Abdominal pain relieved by pressing
- Loose stool
- Copious clear urine
- Shortness of breath and weakness
- Pale tongue
- Feeble or deep slow and weak pulse

Cold Syndrome of Excess Type. Cold syndrome of the excess type is a syndrome due to excessive *yin*-cold inside the body and stagnation of *yang-qi* of *zang-fu* organs. This condition results from an excessive intake of cold or raw food or the direct invasion of the interior by pathogenic cold.

It manifests as:

- Aversion to cold and cold limbs
- Epigastric chilliness and pain
- Abdominal pain and tenderness
- Vomiting watery fluid

- Borborygmus
- Chronic diarrhea
- Cough with profuse thin and whitish sputum
- Asthma
- Whitish slippery fur of the tongue
- Slow or tense pulse

9.5 DIFFERENTIAL DIAGNOSIS OF *YIN* AND *YANG*

Differential diagnosis of *yin* and *yang* is the general guiding principle underlying differential diagnosis by the eight principal syndromes; it governs the other six. For instance, exterior, heat, and excess syndromes are classified into the category of *yang*, while interior, cold, and deficiency syndromes into that of *yin*. The manifestations, etiology, pathogenesis, and treatment of the six principal syndromes have already been dealt with respectively in the previous sections. All diseases can be classified into either *yin* or *yang* according to the pathologic characteristics manifested by clinical syndromes. As stated by Su Wen: "A good doctor first determines the nature of a disease in terms of *yin* and *yang* by observing the complexion and feeling the pulse." However, it must be pointed out that differential diagnosis of *yin* and *yang*, though of great value in the diagnosis of disease, is by no means sufficient for clinical purposes. It has to be employed in combination with other methods of diagnosis, such as differential diagnosis according to the theory of *zang-fu* organs, differential diagnosis according to the theory of *qi*, blood and body fluid, etc.

9.6 DIFFERENTIAL DIAGNOSIS ACCORDING TO THE STATE OF *QI*, BLOOD, AND BODY FLUID

Differential diagnosis according to the state of *qi*, blood, and body fluid is a diagnostic method with which to analyze the pathologic changes and diseases associated with *qi*, blood, and body fluid.

Qi-deficiency Syndrome. *Qi*-deficiency syndrome is a morbid state due to the hypofunction of *zang-fu* organs and general debility due to protracted illness, senile debility, overstrain, and improper diet. It manifests as dizziness, shortness of breath, disinclination to talk, low voice, lassitude, spontaneous perspiration, aggravation of the above symptoms upon exertion, pale tongue, and weak or feeble pulse.

Qi-collapse Syndrome. *Qi*-collapse syndrome refers to a morbid condition of inability of *qi* to rise. Its clinical manifestations are fainting, shortness of breath, lassitude, chronic diarrhea, abdominal distention with tenesmus, prolapsed rectum, prolapsed uterus, weak pulse, and pale tongue with whitish fur. The main characteristics of *qi*-collapse syndrome are symptoms of *qi*-deficiency and ptosis of internal organs.

Qi-stagnation Syndrome. *Qi*-stagnation syndrome refers to a morbid condition due to stagnation of *qi* in a certain locale or organ, resulting from functional disturbance of *zang-fu* organs and disorder of *qi* from emotional upset, improper diet, and invasion by exogenous pathogens. The main clinical manifestations of this syndrome are distention, distress, and pain. *Qi-stagnation* in different locations may give rise to different manifestations. As examples:

- Hypochondriac distending pain accompanied by emotional depression, frequent sighing, and taut pulse marks stagnation of liver-*qi*.
- Stagnation of stomach-*qi* is manifested by epigastric distending pain.
- Stagnation of intestine-*qi* is characterized by abdominal distention and wandering pain.

Syndrome of "Adverseness" of Qi. The syndrome of "adverseness" of *qi* refers to a morbid condition of adverse ascending of *qi* due to its dysfunction. This syndrome primarily indicates functional disturbance of the lungs, stomach, and liver, for it often involves these organs.

- Abnormal ascension of lung-*qi* is manifested as cough and dyspnea.
- Abnormal ascension of stomach-*qi* manifests as hiccups, belching, nausea, and vomiting.
- Abnormal ascension of liver-*qi* manifests as distending pain of the head and eyes, dizziness, or even syncope.

Blood-deficiency Syndrome. Blood-deficiency syndrome refers to a morbid condition due to deficient blood, resulting in failure to nourish *zang-fu* organs and channels. This condition is usually caused by profuse bleeding, weakness and dysfunction of the spleen and stomach, mental overstrain, and consumption of *yin*-fluid. It manifests as pale or sallow complexion, pale lips and nails, dizziness, palpitation, insomnia, numbness of limbs, oligomenorrhea and pale menses, postponed menstrual cycle or menopause, pale tongue, and thready weak pulse.

Blood Stasis Syndrome. Blood stasis syndrome is a morbid condition resulting from the coagulation of blood in a certain region of the body. In this condition, blood is not discharged or dissipated in a timely manner, and stagnation of blood occurs. The common causes of the syndrome are coagulation of cold, stagnation of *qi*, deficient *qi* or trauma. Its clinical manifestations are:

- Localized cutting or stabbing pain aggravated by pressing or at night
- Fullness and tenderness of the abdomen
- Continued bleeding with dark purplish blood, clots or melena
- Dim blackish complexion
- Scaly and dry skin
- Purplish lips and nails
- Capillary congestion or engorged veins visible over the surface of the abdomen
- Varicose veins of the lower limbs with distending pain
- Menopause or dysmenorrhea with dark purplish menses with clots
- Dark purplish tongue or ecchymosis over the tongue
- Hesitant pulse

Blood-heat Syndrome. Blood-heat syndrome refers to spontaneous bleeding due to exuberant heat within the *zang-fu* organs and its attack on *xuefen* (blood system). This condition manifests as bleeding and symptoms indicative of blood heat—such as hematernesis, hemoptysis, hematuria, and hematochezia—all of which show bright red blood, red tongue, and rapid pulse.

Syndrome of Blood Stasis Due to Stagnation of *Qi*. The syndrome of blood stasis due to stagnation of *qi* is primarily related to the dysfunction of the liver caused by emotional upsets. It manifests as symptoms of both *qi*-stagnation and blood stasis, including:

- Restlessness
- Irritability or emotional depression
- Hypochondriac distension and wandering pain
- Distending pain in the breast with masses
- Dysmenorrhea and discharge of dark purplish menses with clots
- Dark purplish tongue or ecchymosis over the tongue
- Hesitant pulse

This syndrome is frequently seen in females.

Deficient *Qi* and Blood. Deficient *qi* and blood refers to the co-existence of *qi*-deficiency and blood-deficiency. This condition is usually caused by an inability of weak *qi* to promote the production of blood or inability of inadequate blood to transform into *qi*. Protracted illness manifests as sallow or pale complexion, dizziness, shortness of breath, disinclination to talk, lassitude, spontaneous perspiration, palpitation, insomnia, pale tongue, and thready, weak pulse.

Syndrome of Blood Loss Due to Deficient *Qi*. The syndrome of loss of blood due to deficient *qi* results in inability to govern blood flow marked by hematemesis, hematochezia, epistaxis, metrorrhagia, lassitude, shortness of breath, pale complexion, pale tongue, and thready, weak pulse.

Syndrome of Massive Hemorrhage Followed by Exhaustion of *Qi*. The syndrome of massive hemorrhage followed by an exhaustion of *qi* refers to a morbid condition of *qi* collapse after sudden massive hemorrhage, usually due to trauma, metrorrhagia, or profuse bleeding after childbirth. This condition manifests as a sudden appearance of pallor during profuse bleeding, cold limbs, profuse perspiration, loss of consciousness, and hollow or indistinct pulse or large but scattered pulse. Clinically, it is often seen in hemorrhagic shock.

Insufficient Body Fluid. Insufficient body fluid leads to its inability to nourish the whole body or some or all of the *zang-fu* organs. Profuse sweating, massive bleeding, severe vomiting, frequent diarrhea, polyuria and consumption of body fluid due to excessive heat usually cause it. Its clinical manifestations are dry mouth and throat, dry or cracked lips, dry or withered skin, dysuria, constipation, red tongue with little saliva and thready, rapid pulse.

Wind-phlegm Syndrome. Wind-phlegm syndrome is provoked by an attack of wind-pathogens. This condition is caused by:

- Wind-*yang* stirring up inside the body due to excess *yang* and deficient *yin*.
- Accumulation of phlegm resulting from excessive intake of fleshy, sweet, and greasy food.

It manifests as dizziness, sudden fainting, wry mouth with distorted eyes, stiff tongue, dysphasia, numbness of the limbs, greasy fur of the tongue, and taut, slippery pulse.

Heat-phlegm Syndrome. Heat-phlegm syndrome results from:
- Production of heat due to accumulation of phlegm-dampness.
- Invasion by *yang*-heat.
- Excess *yang* in the body.
- Transformation of body fluid into phlegm by pathogenic fire that is formed by stagnation of liver-*qi*.

The clinical manifestations of this condition are feverish and restless sensation in the thorax; cough with thick yellowish sputum; dry stool;

inflammation of the throat; yellowish, greasy tongue fur, and rapid, slippery pulse.

Cold-phlegm Syndrome. Cold-phlegm syndrome is caused by abundant expectoration accompanied by cold manifestations. It results from invasion of pathogenic cold and impairment of *yang-qi* or excess *yin* and deficient *yang* leading to stagnation of body fluid with formation of cold-phlegm. Its clinical manifestations are chilliness and cold limbs; whitish, clear and thin phlegm; stabbing pain due to rheumatism involving the bone; inability to raise the limbs; whitish, greasy tongue fur, and deep, slow pulse or deep, slippery pulse.

Damp-phlegm Syndrome. Damp-phlegm syndrome is marked by abundant expectoration accompanied by dampness manifestations. It results from phlegm-dampness due to hypofunction of the spleen. It is also caused by exogenous cold-dampness leading to disturbance of the spleen and stomach—especially dysfunction of the former with phlegm formed from accumulated dampness. Its clinical manifestations are chest oppression and epigastric stuffiness; anorexia; vomiting; nausea; profuse expectoration; heaviness sensation in the limbs; sleepiness; thick, greasy tongue fur, and slippery pulse.

Dry-phlegm Syndrome. Dry-phlegm syndrome results in the production of phlegm from accumulated stool or inflammation of the throat; yellowish, greasy fur of the tongue; and rapid, slippery pulse.

Gastrointestinal Fluid Syndrome. Gastrointestinal fluid syndrome is a morbid condition due to fluid retention in the stomach and intestines. This condition manifests as a full sensation in the chest; splashing sound in the stomach; vomiting clear thin saliva; dizziness; palpitation; shortness of breath; whitish, slippery tongue fur; and taut slippery pulse. It can be seen in gastric retention due to pyloric obstruction, intestinal obstruction due to dropsy and functional disturbance of the stomach and intestines.

Pleural Effusion Syndrome. Pleural effusion syndrome refers to fluid retention in the hypochondrium that manifests as pain over the hypochondriac region. This condition is aggravated by coughing or spitting, dragging pain upon turning over in bed or breathing, fullness sensation over the chest, shortness of breath, and a deep, taut pulse. This syndrome is most often seen in exudative pleuritis.

Anasarca Syndrome. Anasarca syndrome is a morbid condition of accumulated fluid in the subcutaneous tissue. It manifests as heaviness and pain in the limbs, edema, oliguria, fever, aversion to cold, no sweat, cough with frothy sputum, whitish tongue fur, and taut, tense pulse.

Superior-phrenic Fluid Syndrome. Superior-phrenic fluid syndrome is a morbid condition of accumulated excessive fluid above the diaphragm. It manifests as the sensation of oppression in the chest; shortness of breath; difficulty lying on one's back; cough with whitish, frothy sputum; facial edema; whitish, greasy tongue fur, and taut, tense pulse.

9.7 DIFFERENTIAL DIAGNOSIS ACCORDING TO THEORY OF *ZANG-FU* ORGANS

Differential diagnosis according to the theory of the *zang-fu* organs is a diagnostic method based on the analysis and comprehension of symptoms in light of the physiological functions and pathological manifestations of the *zang-fu* organs. This method determines the pathogenesis, nature, and site of a disease and the conflict between body resistance and pathogens as they relate to the *zang-fu* organs.

As an important component of the differential diagnosis system, it serves as the basis of diagnosis for all clinical specialties of TCM. Since the methods of differential diagnosis employed in clinical practice are many and varied, each having its own characteristics, they must first be applied to *zang-fu* organs so as to definitely determine the site and nature of a disease and adopt a treatment accordingly. This method, which lays the foundation for all other methods of differential diagnosis, includes differential diagnosis of *zang* organ diseases, of *fu*-organ diseases, and of diseases of both *zang* and *fu* organs.

Deficient Heart-*qi* or Deficient Heart-*yang* Syndrome. Deficient heart-*qi* and deficient heart-*yang* are due to general asthenia resulting from prolonged illness, consumption of *qi* and impairment of *yang* by sudden onset of a serious illness, visceral dysfunction in the aged, or congenital defects. Deficient heart-*qi* manifests as palpitation, shortness of breath, spontaneous sweating, aggravation of all of the above symptoms upon exertion, pale complexion, lassitude, pale tongue with whitish fur, and weak pulse. Deficient heart-*yang* is marked by all of the symptoms noted above, plus the following symptoms: aversion to cold, cold limbs, dull complexion, pain and oppressed feeling in the pericardial region and flabby, pale, or dark purplish tongue. If symptoms such as profuse sweating, cold limbs, dark purplish lips, weakness of breath, thready and indistinct pulse, delirium, or even unconsciousness are observed, a critical condition of exhausted of heart-*yang* is probable.

Deficient Heart-blood Syndrome or Deficient Heart-*yin* Syndrome. Deficient heart-blood and deficient heart-*yin* are due to:

- Impaired of *yin*-blood by protracted illness
- Profuse blood loss
- Insufficient production of *yin*-blood
- Emotional upsets leading to stagnated *qi* and fire
- Consumption of *yin*-blood.

The main manifestations of heart-blood deficiency syndrome are palpitation, insomnia, frequent dreams, dizziness, poor memory, luster-less complexion, pale lips, pale tongue and thready, weak pulse. In addition to palpitation, insomnia, and poor memory, heart-*yin* deficiency syndrome also manifests as dysphoria with feverish sensation over the palms, soles and the chest; night sweats; dry mouth and throat; reddish tongue with little saliva; and thready, rapid pulse.

Hyperactivity of Heart-fire Syndrome. Hyperactivity of heart-fire syndrome is an interior morbid condition that usually results from production of fire due to:

- Emotional upsets and stagnant *qi*
- Invasion of the interior by the pathogenic fire
- Excessive intake of hot-natured food of acrid taste or warm-natured tonics

This condition manifests as dysphoria with feverish restless sensation in the thorax, insomnia, flushed face, thirst, ulcers of the mouth and tongue, difficult and painful urination with dark urine, hematuria, or mania and delirium, redness of the tip of the tongue, rough and prickle-like tongue fur, and rapid, forceful pulse.

Syndrome of Mental Confusion Due to Phlegm. The syndrome of mental confusion due to phlegm refers to the impairment of consciousness caused by phlegm invading the heart. This condition usually results from the production of phlegm due to emotional upsets and stagnant *qi* or coagulation of the pathogenic dampness in the heart. It manifests as mental depression; apathy; aphrenia; soliloquy; improper behavior; sudden falls with a loss of consciousness; whitish, greasy fur of the tongue; and slippery pulse.

Syndrome of Phlegm-fire Attacking the Heart. The syndrome of phlegm-fire attacking the heart is a morbid condition of mental disturbance due to phlegm-fire. It is caused by emotional upsets, mental depression, and anger leading to stagnation of *qi* and production of fire that transforms fluid into phlegm. It is also caused when pathogenic heat invades the heart converting fluid into phlegm. Its clinical manifestations are fever; raucous breathing; flushed face; congested eyes; expectoration of yellowish, thick phlegm; delirium; red tongue with yellowish, greasy fur; slippery, rapid pulse; insomnia; irritability; profuse sputum; feeling of oppression in the chest; dizziness or paraphasia, and manifestations of mania.

- If the syndrome is caused by invasion by the pathogenic heat, the chief signs for differential diagnosis are high fever, abundant expectoration, and unconsciousness.
- If the syndrome is brought about by internal injury, the main symptoms for diagnosing mild cases are restlessness and insomnia and for diagnosing severe cases, mania.

Syndrome of Stagnated Heart-blood. The syndrome of stagnation of heart-blood is a morbid condition due to obstruction of the heart's collaterals. It results from insufficient heart-*qi* or heart-*yang* or coagulation of phlegm that obstructs the collaterals, and it manifests as:

- Palpitation
- Intermittent choking sensation
- Stabbing pain in the chest
- Dragging pain over the shoulder, back, and arm
- Dark purplish tongue perhaps with petechiae and ecchymosis
- Small, hesitant pulse or slow, weak pulse with irregular intervals

In severe cases of this syndrome, a sudden attack of intolerable pain, cyanosis of the mouth, lips and nails, cold limbs, coma and faint, indistinct pulse occurs.

Syndrome of Deficient Lung-*qi*. Deficient lung-*qi* results from the lungs' hypofunction, usually resulting from impaired lung-*qi* due to protracted illness and/or insufficient *qi*-production. It is marked by cough with dyspnea; shortness of breath aggravated on slight exertion; clear, thin sputum; low, weak voice; pale complexion; lassitude; spontaneous perspiration; aversion to wind; susceptibility to cold due to exogenous pathogens; pale tongue with whitish fur; and feeble pulse.

Syndrome of Deficient Lung-*yin*. Deficient lung-*qi* indicates insufficient lung-*yin* and the production of heat deficiency inside the body. This condition usually results from impaired *yin* by prolonged cough, injury of the lungs by pathogens or impairment of *yin*-fluid in the late stage of a febrile disease. It is marked by:

- Dry cough with no sputum or with scanty viscid sputum
- Dry mouth and throat
- Emaciation
- Afternoon fever

- Dysphoria with feverish sensation in the chest, palms, and soles
- Flushed cheeks and/or night sweats
- Bloody sputum
- Reddish tongue with little fur
- Thready, rapid pulse

Syndrome of Wind-cold Pathogen Tightening the Lungs.
When the wind-cold pathogen tightens the lungs, lung-*qi* is obstructed. This condition manifests as a cough with whitish thin sputum, stuffy nose with watery discharge, slight aversion to cold, mild fever, no sweat, whitish tongue fur, and floating, tense pulse.

Syndrome of Cold Pathogen Attacking the Lungs. When cold pathogen attacks the lungs, it manifests as a cough with dyspnea and thin whitish sputum, chilliness and cold limbs, pale tongue with whitish fur, and slow or moderated pulse.

Syndrome of Retained Pathogenic Heat in the Lungs. When pathogenic heat is retained in the lungs, it causes dysfunction of lung-*qi* and is usually caused by the pathogenic heat attacking the lungs or accumulated of heat in the lungs converted from wind-cold or wind-heat resulting from *yang*-excess. Its clinical manifestations are dyspnea, cough with thick yellowish sputum, high fever, thirst, irritability, flaring of nares, chest pain, blood and pus-stained sputum with stinking smell, constipation, scanty dark urine, reddish tongue with yellowish fur, and slippery rapid pulse.

Syndrome of Attack of the Lungs by Pathogenic Dryness.
When pathogenic dryness attacks the lungs, they are impaired by fluid in autumn. This condition manifests as:

- Dry cough with no sputum or with scanty viscid sputum difficult to expectorate
- Chest pain due to violent cough
- Dry mouth, lips, nose, and throat
- Fever
- Slight aversion to wind and cold
- Thin, dry fur of the tongue
- Thready, rapid pulse

Syndrome of Accumulated Phlegm-dampness in the Lungs.
When phlegm-dampness accumulates in the lungs, it stagnates in the pulmonary system and usually results from impaired dispersing and descending function of the lungs. This condition results when pathogenic cold and dampness attacks or when phlegm-dampness accumu-

lates. Usually, protracted cough and stagnated phlegm in the lungs transforms from water-dampness impairs the lungs. This is due to spleen-*qi*'s inability to transport body fluids. The clinical manifestations of this condition are cough with copious whitish and thin sputum that is easily expectorated, feeling of oppression in the chest, dyspnea, pale tongue with whitish greasy fur, taut and slippery or soft and floating pulse.

Syndrome of Damp-heat in the Large Intestine. Damp-heat is retained in the large intestine because of an affection by the exogenous damp-heat pathogen or because one has consumed unclean food. The clinical manifestations of this condition are:

- Abdominal pain
- Diarrhea with purulent and bloody stool
- Tenesmus or sudden onset of diarrhea with discharge of yellowish, stinking stool accompanied by burning sensation in the anus
- Dry mouth without the desire to drink
- Scanty dark urine
- Fever with or without aversion to cold
- Red tongue with greasy, yellowish fur
- Soft and rapid or slippery and rapid pulse

Syndrome of Deficient Fluid in the Large Intestine. Deficient fluid in the large intestine results mainly from a *yin* deficiency in the aged, chronic disease consuming *yin*, consumption of body fluid by febrile disease, or hemorrhage after delivery in women. Its clinical manifestation are constipation (even one bowel movement in several days); dry mouth and throat; dry, red tongue; thready and hesitant pulse; halitosis and dizziness.

Syndrome of Insufficient Spleen-*qi*. The spleen's inability to transport or transform nutrients due to insufficient spleen-*qi* is usually caused by:

- Improper diet
- Fatigue
- Internal injury
- Other acute of chronic disorders that consume spleen-*qi*

Its clinical manifestations are poor appetite, abdominal distention aggravated after meals, diarrhea or loose stool, sallow complexion, shortness of breath, disinclination to talk due to mental fatigue, lassitude of limbs, pale tongue with whitish fur, and slow, weak pulse.

Syndrome of Deficient Spleen-*yang*. Deficient spleen-*yang* is a syndrome of overabundance of *yin*-cold due to insufficient spleen-*yang*, resulting from insufficient spleen-*qi* or from excessive intake of raw or cold food or cold-natured medicine, which injures spleen-*yang*. The clinical manifestations of this condition are:

- Abdominal distention, poor appetite, and abdominal pain relieved by pressing
- Preference for warmth
- Clear, thin, and loose stool
- Cold limbs
- Profuse, thin leukorrhea
- Pale and swollen tongue with whitish glossy fur
- Deep, slow and weak pulse

Syndrome of Collapsed Spleen-*qi*. Collapse of spleen-*qi* is a syndrome marked by the inability of spleen-*qi* to rise. This condition results mostly from dysfunctional spleen-*qi*, from chronic diarrhea and dysentery, or from overstrains. Its clinical manifestations are:

- Distention and bearing down sensation of the epigastrium aggravated after eating meat
- Tenesmus of the anus
- Chronic diarrhea or dysentery
- Prolapse of the rectum and uterus

This condition is often accompanied with shortness of breath, disinclination to talk, lassitude, dizziness, and pale tongue with whitish fur and weak pulse.

Syndrome of the Spleen's Failure to Control Blood Flow. Failure of the spleen to control blood flow is a syndrome marked by the inability of the spleen to keep blood flowing within the vessels due to insufficient spleen-*qi*. This condition is mainly caused by injury to the spleen due to chronic disease or fatigue. Its clinical manifestation are hemafecia, metrorrhagia, metrostaxis, hematuria, hematohidrosis, and gingival hemorrhage; these symptoms are often accompanied by:

- Lassitude
- Shortness of breath
- Disinclination to talk
- Poor appetite
- Loose stool
- Pale complexion

- Pale tongue with whitish fur
- Thready, weak pulse

Syndrome of Retained Cold and Dampness in the Spleen. The retention of cold and dampness in the spleen is attributed to excessive cold and dampness in the body and impaired *yang* of the middle-*jiao*. This syndrome is due to the following:
- Excessive intake of raw or unripe fruits
- Exposure to cold
- Preference for cold drinks
- Exposure to wetness because of braving the rain or wading across rivers
- Cold and damp living conditions
- Cold and dampness accumulated in the body

The clinical manifestations of this condition are:
- Eigastric distention and stuffiness
- Poor appetite
- Nausea
- Flat taste in the mouth
- No thirst
- Abdominal pain
- Loose stool
- Heavy sensation in the head and body
- Dim yellow complexion
- Edema of the limbs
- Oliguria
- Pale, swollen tongue with whitish and greasy fur
- Soft, slow pulse

Syndrome of Retained Damp-heat in the Spleen. The retention of damp-heat in the spleen is attributed to the accumulation of pathogenic damp-heat in the middle-*jiao*, which results from an attack by exogenous pathogenic damp-heat and excessive intake of fatty, sweet, and greasy food. Its clinical manifestations are:
- Abdominal distention, poor appetite, and nausea
- Loose stool and yellowish urine
- Heavy sensation in the limbs
- Bright orange complexion of the skin and sclera
- Irregular paroxysm of fever that profuse sweating does not relieve

- Red tongue with yellowish and greasy fur
- Soft, rapid pulse

Syndrome of Stomach-cold. Stomach-cold is due to stagnation of pathogenic cold in the stomach, usually caused by improper mode of living, exposure of the abdomen to cold, or excessive intake of raw or cold food. Its clinical manifestations are:

- Cold-pain in the epigastrium and abdomen—mild or severe, but relieved by warmth and aggravated by cold
- Flat taste in the mouth and an absence of thirst
- Rumbling in the stomach
- Salivation and a whitish, slippery fur of the tongue
- Slow or taut pulse

In the case of repeated and protracted attacks of the disorder with resultant damage of the *yang-qi*, such symptoms as lassitude, listlessness, cold limbs with desire for warmth and others are likely to ensue.

Syndrome of Stomach-heat. Stomach-heat is a syndrome of excessive pathogenic heat in the stomach, caused by invasion of pathogenic fire that results from excessive intake of acrid, fatty and sweet food, stagnated *qi* or of emotional depression. Its clinical manifestations are:

- Burning pain in the epigastrium and gastric discomfort with acid regurgitation
- Thirst with desire for cold drinks
- Halitosis
- Vomiting immediately after meals,
- Polyorexia
- Inflamed, ulcerated or bleeding gums
- Constipation and/or scanty dark urine
- Red tongue with yellowish fur
- Slippery and rapid pulse

Syndrome of Retention of Undigested Food in the Stomach.
Indigestion is usually due to immoderate eating and drinking. Its clinical manifestations include:

- Epigastric distention and stuffiness or pain
- Belching with foul taste and smell
- Vomiting acid and rotten food with distention and pain relieved after vomiting
- Flatulence and loose stool with acid, rotten and foul smells

- Thick and greasy fur on the tongue
- Slippery pulse

Syndrome of Deficient Stomach-yin. Deficient stomach-*yin* results from failure of *yin*-fluid to be restored after prolonged febrile disease or impairment of stomach-*yin* by excessive intake of pungent food. Its clinical manifestations are dull pain of the epigastrium, hunger with disinclination to eat, belching, hiccups, dry mouth and throat, constipation, red tongue with thin dry fur and thready, rapid pulse.

Syndrome of Stagnated Liver-*qi*. Stagnation of liver-*qi* is characterized by an inability of the liver to disperse *qi*. It usually results from emotional depression, abrupt mental irritation and invasion by other pathogens. Its clinical manifestations are:

- Emotional depression and irritability
- Stuffiness in the chest
- Frequent sighing
- Wandering pain with distension in the chest, hypochondrium and lower abdomen
- Sensation of a foreign body in the throat which cannot be swallowed or coughed up
- Goiter and/or abdominal mass

Additionally, women may experience distending pain in breasts, dysmenorrhea and irregular menstruation, whitish fur on the tongue, and taut pulse.

Syndrome of Flaring-up of the Liver-fire. An adverse rising of *qi* and fire from the liver marks the syndrome in which the liver-fire flares up. It results mostly from an attack of fire due to emotional upsets; stagnation of liver-*qi*; excessive intake of acrid, fatty and sweet food and transformation of accumulated heat into fire. Its clinical manifestations are:

- Dizziness
- Distending headache and flushed face
- Conjunctival congestion
- Bitter taste and a dry mouth
- Restlessness and irritability, insomnia and nightmares
- Burning pain in the hypochondrium
- Constipation and dark urine
- Tinnitus, otopyorrhea, hematemesis, and epistaxis
- Red tongue with yellow fur
- Taut, rapid pulse

Syndrome of Deficient Liver-blood. Deficient liver-blood is due to dysfunction in both the spleen and kidneys, massive loss of blood, or consumption of liver-blood because of chronic disorders. Its clinical manifestations are:

- Pallor
- Dizziness and tinnitus
- Dryness and discomfort of the eyes, poor sight and night blindness
- Numbness of the limbs
- Contraction of tendons and muscles and/or muscular twitching
- Colorless nails
- Pale tongue
- Thready, taut pulse

Additionally, women may also experience scanty, light-colored menstrual discharge or even amenorrhea.

Syndrome of Deficient Liver-*yin*. Deficient liver-*yin* is a syndrome of deficient *yin*-fluid of the liver that results primarily from fire transformed from stagnated liver-*qi* due to emotional upsets or impaired liver-*yin* in a prolonged liver disorder or febrile disease in the late stages. It manifests clinically as:

- Dizziness and/or tinnitus
- Dryness and discomfort of the eyes
- Feeling of extreme heat on the face
- Distention of or burning pains in the hypochondrium
- Dyspharia with feverish sensation in the chest, palms and soles
- Hectic fever and/or night sweats
- Dry mouth and throat
- Involuntary movement of the limbs
- Red and dry tongue
- Thready, taut and rapid pulse

Syndrome of Hyperactive Liver-*yang*. The syndrome of hyperactivity of the liver-*yang* is caused by deficient *yin*-fluid in the liver and the kidneys. (Remember, that in this case, the kidney-water fails to moisten the liver-wood.) This condition results mostly from liver-fire due to anger and anxiety, stagnation of liver-*qi*, consumption of *yin*-fluid, and failure of *yin* to counterbalance *yang*. Its clinical manifestations are:

- Dizziness, vertigo, and/or tinnitus
- Distending pain in the head and eyes
- Flushed face and conjunctival congestion
- Irritability and palpitation
- Amnesia, insomnia, and/or dreaminess
- Weakness of the loins and knees
- Red tongue
- Taut forceful pulse or thready, taut and rapid pulse

Syndrome of Up-Stirring of the Liver-wind. Stirring up the liver-wind is a morbid condition clinically manifested as dizziness leading to falls, tremors, and convulsions.

Generally, the following three types are recognized:

1. Syndrome of interior wind transformed from the liver-*yang* is a syndrome due to failure to suppress the hyperactive liver-*yang*. Its clinical manifestations are a tendency to fall from dizziness, head-shaking due to distending pain, stiff neck, tremor, aphasia, numbness of the limbs, abnormal gait or sudden syncope, unconsciousness, facial distortion, hemiplegia, red and stiff tongue and taut, forceful pulse or thready, taut and rapid pulse.

2. Syndrome of interior wind resulting from over-abundance of heat is a syndrome occurring in the case of extreme hyperactivity of pathogenic heat. Its clinical manifestations are high fever, coma, restlessness, convulsion of the limbs, stiff neck, eyeballs turning upwards, lockjaw or opisthotonos, red or crimson tongue, and taut, rapid pulse.

3. Syndrome of interior wind caused by deficient blood is a morbid condition due to lack of nourishment to the tendons and muscles owing to deficient blood stored in the liver. For clinical manifestations refer to the section Syndrome of Deficient Liver-blood, page 170.

Syndrome of Dampness and Heat in the Liver and the Gallbladder. Dampness and heat in the liver and gallbladder is a morbid condition due to:

- Exogenous damp-heat pathogen
- Excessive intake of fatty, sweet, and indigestible food
- Accumulation of pathogenic dampness in the body that is transformed into heat due to the spleen's dysfunction when performing its transporting function

Its clinical manifestations include:
- Distending pain in the hypochondrium or abdominal mass
- Anorexia
- Abdominal distention
- Bitter taste
- Nausea
- Abnormal stool
- Scanty, dark urine
- Red tongue with yellowish, greasy fur
- Taut and rapid pulse
- Alternate attacks of chills and fever
- Eczema of the scrotum with intolerable itching
- Swollen testes with a sensation of pain and heat
- Foul and yellowish leukorrhea

Syndrome of Accumulated Cold in the Liver Channel. Cold, accumulated in the liver channel is due to pathogenic cold invading the liver. Its clinical manifestations are:
- Cold pain in the lower abdomen
- Bearing down or distending pain in the testes
- Dragging pain in the scrotum upon contraction, aggravated by cold and relieved by heat
- and glossy fur on the tongue
- Deep and taut or slow pulse

Syndrome of Phlegm Attack Due to Stagnated Gallbladder-*qi*. When the gallbladder fails to properly disperse gallbladder-*qi*, the gallbladder-*qi* stagnates and phlegm attacks the body. This morbid condition results mainly from emotional upsets, depressed *qi*, and the gallbladder's failure to perform its dispersing function. Its clinical manifestations are:
- Palpitation
- Insomnia and restlessness
- Stuffiness in the chest and distented the hypochondrium
- Bitter taste
- Nausea and dizziness
- Yellow and greasy fur on the tongue
- Taut slippery pulse

Syndrome of Deficient Kidney-*yang*. Deficient kidney-*yang* results mainly from kidney-dysfunction in the aged, kidney injury due to chronic disorders and intemperance in sexual life. The clinical manifestations of this condition are:

- Pallor
- Aversion to cold and cold limbs
- Listless, weakness, or cold-pain in the loins and knees
- Impotence in men and sterility in women due to cold womb
- Persistent diarrhea with undigested food in the stool or diarrhea before dawn
- Edema (more serious in lower limbs)
- Pale and swollen tongue with whitish coating
- Deep, thready and weak pulse (more obvious in the *chi* position of the pulse)

Syndrome of Deficient Kidney-*yin*. Deficient kidney-*yin* is due to insufficient *yin*-fluid in the kidneys. This condition results mainly from kidney injury due to chronic disorders, intemperance in sexual life, and excessive intake of acrid, dry food, which leads to consumption of *yin*. Its clinical manifestations are:

- Weakness of the loins and knees
- Dizziness and/or tinnitus
- Insomnia and dreaminess
- Tidal fever and/or night sweats
- Dysphoria with feverish sensation in the chest, palms and soles
- Flushed cheeks and dry throat
- Emaciation
- Constipation
- Pale tongue with little fur
- Thready, rapid pulse
- Frequent erection of the penis or emission in men
- Scanty menstruation or amenorrhea in women

Syndrome of "Unconsolidation" of Kidney-*qi*. The kidney inability to consolidate kidney-*qi* is a morbid condition due to decreased renal function. This condition usually results from kidney-deficiency in the aged, insufficient kidney-*qi* in infants, chronic disorders consuming kidney-*qi*, or intemperance in sexual life. Its clinical manifestations are:

- Lassitude and listlessness
- Weakness of the loins and knees
- Frequent micturition with light-colored urine
- Urinary incontinence and/or continuous dripping after urination or enuresis
- Pale tongue with whitish fur
- Deep weak pulse
- Nocturia, spermatorrhea or premature ejaculation in men
- Clear leukorrhea or spontaneous abortion in women

Syndrome of Insufficient Kidney-essence. Consumption of kidney-essence is caused mainly by congenital defects, improper care after birth, intemperance in sexual life, and injury of the kidneys due to chronic disorders. Its clinical manifestations are:
- In infants: retarded development, marked by microsoma, low intelligence, bradypragia, tardy closure of fontanel, and dysostosis
- In adults, sterility due to spermacrasia in males and due to amenorrhea in females, premature senility, baldness and odonteseisis, tinnitus, deafness, amnesia, trance, flaccidity of feet, hyponea, and bradypragia

Syndrome of Damp-heat in the Urinary Bladder. The retention of pathogenic damp-heat in the urinary bladder usually results from immoderate diet. Its clinical manifestations are frequent and urgent micturition; scanty, brownish-red, cloudy urine; fever and lumbago; red tongue with yellowish and greasy fur; and slippery, rapid pulse.

Syndrome of Breakdown of the Normal Physiological Coordination between the Heart and Kidneys. This is a morbid condition attributable to a lack of coordination between water (the kidneys) and fire (the heart). It results mainly from consumption of kidney-*yin* due to chronic disorders, intemperance in sexual life, and production of fire due to over-anxiety or emotional depression.

Its clinical manifestations are:
- Vexation, insomnia, and/or palpitation
- Dizziness and/or tinnitus
- Amnesia
- Soreness of the waist and knees
- Seminal emission
- Dysphoria with feverish sensation in the chest, palms and soles

- Dry throat and mouth
- Red tongue
- Thready and rapid pulse

These symptoms are sometimes accompanied by lassitude and feeling of cold in the loins and knees.

Syndrome of Deficient *Yang* in the Heart and Kidneys.
Deficient *yang* in the heart and kidneys indicates either insufficient *yang-qi* in the heart and the kidneys or overabundant *yin*-cold pathogens in the body. This condition results mainly from protracted illness or internal injury due to overstrain. Its clinical manifestations are: aversion to cold and cold limbs; palpitation; dysuria; edema in the face and lower limbs; cyanotic lips and nails; pale, dark and cyanotic tongue with whitish and glossy fur and deep, thready and feeble pulse.

Syndrome of Deficient *Qi* in the Heart and Lungs. This is a morbid condition due to insufficient heart-*qi* and lung-*qi*. It is usually brought about by overstrain or consumption of *qi* in the heart and the lungs due to chronic cough with dyspnea. Its clinical manifestations are:

- Palpitation and shortness of breath
- Cough with dyspnea
- Thoracic stuffiness
- Weakness with spontaneous sweating especially upon exertion
- Pallor or dark complexion or even cyanotic lips
- Pale tongue with whitish fur
- Thready, weak pulse

Syndrome of Deficient *Qi* in the Lungs and Kidneys.
Insufficient lung-*qi* and kidney-*qi* usually results from consumption of lung-*qi* and injury of the kidney-*qi* by cough with dyspnea due to protracted illness. Its clinical manifestations are:

- Dyspnea, sometimes severe
- Shortness of breath with prolonged exhalation and shortened inhalation
- Difficulty in breathing, more obvious upon exertion
- Spontaneous sweating
- Lassitude
- Weakness of the lions and knees
- Pale tongue with whitish coating

- Deep and weak pulse
- Cold limbs
- Cyanotic complexion and severe clammy sweating
- Floating, large, unrooted pulse (easily felt on light pressure but disappearing on heavy pressure)

Syndrome of Deficient *Yin* in the Lungs and Kidneys.
Insufficient *yin*-fluid in both the lungs and the kidneys results in:
- Consumption of lung-*yin* due to chronic cough, leading to deficient lungs and affecting the kidneys
- Injury of kidney-*yin* due to protracted illness or excess sexual intercourse, thus leading to deficient kidneys and involving the lungs

The clinical manifestations of this condition are:
- Cough with scanty sputum or blood-tinged sputum
- Dry throat and mouth and hoarseness
- Emaciation and weakness of the lions and knees
- Hectic and regular recurrent fever, flushed cheeks, and night sweats
- Red tongue with little fur
- Thready, rapid pulse
- Seminal emission in males
- Irregular menstruation in females

Syndrome of Deficient *Yin* in the Liver and Kidneys.
Insufficient *yin*-fluid in both the liver and the kidneys is most often a result of the consumption of essense and blood. This condition is due to intemperance in sexual life, internal injury by the seven emotions, or consumption of *yin* in both the liver and the kidneys due to protracted illness. The clinical manifestations of this condition are:
- Dizziness and tinnitus resembling the sound of a cicada
- Dull pain in the hypochondium
- Amnesia
- Insomnia
- Weakness of the loins and knees
- Dry throat and mouth
- Dysphoria with feverish sensation in the chest, palms, and soles
- Flushed cheeks and night sweats
- Red tongue with little fur

- Thready rapid pulse
- Seminal emission in males
- Scanty menstruation in females

Syndrome of Deficient *Yang* in the Spleen and Kidneys.
Insufficient spleen-*yang* and kidney-*yang* results from:
- Consumption of *yang* and *qi* due to chronic disorders of the spleen and the kidneys
- Failure to warm and nourish spleen-*yang* due to chronic diarrhea, dysentery, and persistent stagnation of water pathogen
- Failure to fill and nourish kidney-*yang* due to chronic deficient spleen-*yang*

The clinical manifestations of this condition include:
- Pallor
- Aversion to cold; cold limbs; and feeling of cold-pain in the waist, knees and lower abdomen
- Chronic diarrhea and dysentery, diarrhea before dawn, or diarrhea with undigested food in the stool
- Dysuria
- Puffy face and edema of the limbs
- Severe abdominal distention resembling the shape of a drum
- Pale and swollen tongue with whitish and glossy fur
- Deep, weak pulse

Syndrome of Deficient *Qi* in the Spleen and Lungs. Deficient spleen-*qi* and lung-*qi* usually results from:
- Improper function the lungs due to chronic cough with dyspnea, which, in turn, affects the spleen.
- Injury of the spleen due to improper diet and overstrain leading to its failure to transport essence to the lungs.

Its clinical manifestations are protracted cough, shortness of breath with dyspnea, expectoration of profuse clear sputum, poor appetite, abdominal distention, loose stool, lassitude, debility with disinclination to talk, pallor or even puffiness of face and feet, pale tongue with whitish fur, and thready, weak pulse.

Syndrome of a Lack of Coordination between the Liver and Spleen. The inability to properly coordinate the efforts of the liver and spleen is the result of stagnated liver-*qi* and dysfunction of the spleen in transport. This condition stems from:

- Liver impairment due to emotional upsets and enduring anger leading to dysfunction of the liver, which, in turn, affects the spleen's transport function.
- Spleen impairment from improper diet and overstrain leading to its deficiency, which, in turn, gives rise to stagnation of pathogenic dampness in the body and affects the liver's function.

Its clinical manifestations are distending and wandering pain in the chest and hypochondrium, sighing, emotional stress, irritability, poor appetite, abdominal distention, loose stool, borborygmus, flatulence, abdominal pain relieved after diarrhea, whitish fur on the tongue, and taut pulse.

Syndrome of a Lack of Coordination between the Liver and Stomach. The inability to coordinate the functions of the liver and stomach is indicative of dysfunction of both the liver and the stomach. It usually results from emotional depression and the stagnation of hyperactive liver-*qi* attacking the stomach. Its clinical manifestations are:

- Chest stuffiness
- Distention and pain in the hypochondriac region and the epigastrium
- Hiccups, belching, and gastric discomfort with acid regurgitation
- Anxiety and irritability
- Whitish, yellowish, and thin fur on the tongue
- Taut pulse

Syndrome of Deficient *Qi* and Blood in the Heart and Spleen. Characterized by insufficient heart-blood and deficient spleen-*qi*, this syndrome results mainly from improper care after protracted illness, worries, fatigue, and chronic hemorrhage. Its clinical manifestations are:
- Palpitation
- Insomnia and dreaminess
- Dizziness
- Amnesia
- Sallow complexion and poor appetite
- Abdominal distention and loose stool
- Lassitude and weakness
- Subcutaneous hemorrhage
- Pale and tender tongue

- Thready weak pulse
- Scanty light-colored menstruation for a prolonged period in women

Syndrome of Invasion of the Lungs by the Liver-fire. This is a syndrome due to upward invasion of the lungs by the *qi* and fire in the liver leading to pulmonary dysfunction in purification and descent. Fire invades the lungs because liver-*qi* stagnates—due to either emotional depression or pathogenic heat invading the liver—and rises to the lungs. Its clinical manifestations are:
- Burning pain in the chest and hypochondrium
- Irritability
- Dizziness
- Conjunctival congestion
- Dysphoria with a smothering sensation
- Bitter taste
- Paroxysmal cough or hemoptysis
- Red tongue with yellow, thin fur
- Taut rapid pulse

9.8 DIFFERENTIAL DIAGNOSIS IN ACCORDANCE WITH THE THEORY OF SIX CHANNELS

This is one of the methods of differential diagnosis for exopathic diseases, put forward by Zhang Zhongjing, a distinguished physician in the Han dynasty. In accordance with the general guiding principle of *yin* and *yang*, this theory divides all of the symptoms and signs appearing in exopathic diseases into two main categories: diseases of the three *yang* channels and diseases of the three *yin* channels.

According to their nature, diseases of three *yang* channels can be further divided into *taiyang* disease, *yangming* disease, and *shaoyang* disease. Those of the three *yin* channels are categorized as *taiyin* disease, *shaoyin* disease, and *jueyin* disease. The six channel diseases are manifestations of the pathologic changes in *zang-fu* organs, channels, and collaterals. The pathologic changes of the six *fu* organs are the dominant factors in diseases of three *yang* channels, and those of the five *zang* organs are dominant in diseases of the three *yin* channels. This theory reveals to some extent the laws governing the development and changes of exopathic diseases.

Syndromes of *Taiyang* Disease. The *taiyang* channels, which serve as a fence protecting the human body, dominate the skin and muscles and govern nutritive *qi* and defensive *qi*. Dysfunction of defensive *qi* due to invasion of the skin and muscles by exogenous pathogens is called *taiyang* disease, whose main symptoms and signs are fever, aversion to cold, rigidity of the nape with headache, and floating pulse.

- When exogenous pathogens invade the body, the defensive *qi* goes to the skin to resist them and a conflict between the vital *qi* (defensive *qi*) and the pathogens ensues, thereby leading to fever.

- Since the defensive *qi* is consumed on the skin, it fails to warm the body and the symptom of aversion to cold appears.

- As the defensive-*qi* stimulates the pulse to the exterior it feels floating.

- The channel of foot-*taiyang* originates from the inner canthus, goes up to the forehead and then to the vertex, where it turns back into the head to link with the brain and then goes down along the nape and back. When exogenous pathogens invade the body, the channel ceases to function properly and the symptom of rigidity of the nape with headache occurs.

Depending on the nature of exogenous pathogens and the patient's constitution, *taiyang* disease can be classified into two types: *taiyang* wind-affection syndrome and *taiyang* cold-stroke syndrome.

Taiyang **Wind-affection Syndrome.** Because of the skin's lowered resistance, when wind-pathogen attacks the body perspiration appears due to the striae's loosening. Other symptoms such as fever, aversion to wind, headache and floating, moderate pulse may appear.

Taiyang Cold-stroke Syndrome. The morbid condition in which the striae of the skin and muscles close when pathogenic cold attacks the body is known as *Taiyang* cold-stroke syndrome. During this condition, no perspiration occurs and symptoms such as fever, aversion to cold, rigidity of the nape with headache, general aching, anhidrosis, dyspnea, and floating and tense pulse appear.

Syndrome of *Yangming* Disease. *Yangming* disease is regarded as an interior heat syndrome that shows as lesions on the skin. Because of erroneous treatment of *taiyang* disease, the pathogens entering the interior of the body convert into heat, which not only consumes body fluid, but also produces pathogenic dryness. This, in turn, accumulates to produce excess syndrome. The exopathogens attacking the body may also turn into heat due to the body's hyperactivity *yang*. According to the location of the lesion and characteristics of the symptoms and signs, *yangming* diseases can be classified as either *yangming* channel syndrome or *yangming fu*-organ syndrome.

Yangming Channel Syndrome. Characterized by overabundance of heat in the *yangming* channel, this syndrome allows no stercoroma in the intestinal tract despite pathogenic heat's spreading throughout all parts of the body. Its clinical manifestations include high fever, profuse sweating, extreme thirst, full and large pulse, dysphoria, flushed face, and yellow, dry fur on the tongue. *Yangming Fu*-organ Syndrome

This is a morbid condition of formation of stercoroma in the intestinal tract as a result of combination and accumulation of pathogenic heat and stool. Its clinical manifestations are:

Afternoon fever

- Panhidrosis or polyhidrosis of hands and feet
- Abdominal distension with pain and tenderness
- Constipation of solid fecal material in the large intestinal tract or watery stool with a foul smell
- Restlessness
- Delirium
- Yellow, thick, and dry fur on the tongue or even burnt black, fissured and prickly tongue
- Deep, slow and forceful pulse

Syndrome of *Shaoyang* Disease. *Shaoyang* disease is a morbid condition with the pathogens located in the half-skin/half-interior of the body. Its clinical manifestations are bitter taste in the mouth, dry throat, dizziness, sensation of pain and fullness in the chest and hypochondrium, alternate attacks of chills and fever, poor appetite, vexation, vomiting, whitish or thin and yellowish fur on the tongue; and taut pulse.

Syndrome of *Taiyin* Disease. *Taiyin* is an interior cold syndrome of the deficiency type brought about by insufficient spleen-*yang*. Its clinical manifestations are abdominal fullness, vomiting, anorexia, diarrhea, no thirst, frequent abdominal pain, whitish fur on the tongue, and weak, moderate pulse.

Syndrome of *Shaoyin* Disease. *Shaoyin* disease is a syndrome due to the hypofunction of the heart and the kidneys, which are the viscera of fire and water, respectively, and the sources of *yin* and *yang*. The invasion of the exopathogens on the *shaoyin* channel results in the hypofunction of the heart and the kidneys characterized by excess *yin* due to *yang* insufficiency or hyperactivity of fire due to *yin* deficiency. The former indicates cold syndrome of *shaoyin*, while the latter, its heat syndrome. However, as far as exogenous febrile diseases are concerned, cold syndrome of *shaoyin* occurs more frequently than heat syndrome.

Cold Syndrome of *Shaoyin*. Cold syndrome of *shaoyin* disease refers to a systemic asthenia-cold syndrome due to the hypofunction of *yang-qi* in the heart and the kidneys. Its clinical manifestations are aversion to cold, curling up during sleep, listlessness, cold limbs, diarrhea with undigested food in the stool, poor appetite, vomiting after meals, and faint indistinct pulse.

Heat Syndrome of *Shaoyin*. Heat syndrome of *shaoyin* disease is a syndrome of deficient genuine *yin* and kidney-fluid. Its clinical manifestations are vexation, insomnia, dry throat and mouth, reddish tongue tip or crimson tongue with little fur, and thready, rapid pulse.

Syndrome of *Jueyin* Disease. The *jueyin* channel lies at the end of *yin* and the beginning of *yang*. *Jueyin* disease is a morbid condition caused by pathogens attacking the *jueyin* channel, leading to exhaustion of vital *qi* of the body and imbalance between *yin* and *yang*. This condition is characterized by simultaneous occurrence of cold and heat syndromes and alternate attacks of chills and fever. Its clinical manifestations are persistent thirst, upward reflux of gas, chest pain with hot sensation, hunger with no desire for eating, cold limbs, diarrhea, vomiting or even vomiting of ascaris, and alternate spells of chills and fever.

9.9 DIFFERENTIAL DIAGNOSIS BY THE ANALYSIS OF *WEIQI, YING,* AND *XUE*

Ye Tianshi, an eminent physician of the Qing dynasty developed a diagnostic method for epidemic febrile diseases by exopathogens and analysis of *weiqi, ying,* and *xue*. His theory was founded on the basis of differential diagnosis in accordance with the theory of six channels and served as a supplement to that theory. The differential diagnosis by the analysis of *weiqi, ying,* and *xue* classifies all intricate clinical manifestations in epidemic febrile diseases into four categories: *weifen, qifen, yingfen* and *xuefen* syndromes, which denote the four different stages (superficial, deep, mild and serious) in the development of an epidemic febrile disease.

***Weifen* Syndrome.** *Weifen* syndrome occurs when warm-heat pathogens attack the superficies of the body and defensive *qi* ceases to function properly. It is mostly seen at the initial stage of an epidemic febrile disease. Its clinical manifestations are fever, slight aversion to wind and cold, headache, dry mouth, slight thirst, cough, swollen and sore throat, red tip and edge of the tongue, and floating rapid pulse.

***Qifen* Syndrome.** *Qifen* syndrome is a syndrome of internal heat due to overabundance of heat caused by:
- Invasion of the interior of the body from the superficies by the pathogenic heat.

- Sharp conflict between the undiminished vital *qi* and excessive pathogens.

Its clinical manifestations are fever, aversion to heat rather than cold, red tongue with yellowish fur, and rapid pulse. Vexation, thirst, and scanty, dark urine often accompany these symptoms. Additional symptoms may be exhibited as follows:

- In the case of stagnation of the pathogenic heat in the lungs: cough or cough with yellowish thick sputum, dyspnea, and chest pain.
- In the case of affection of the chest and diaphragm by the pathogenic heat: vexation, heartburn, and restlessness.
- In the case of invasion of the stomach by the pathogenic heat: high fever, profuse sweating, extreme thirst, and large full pulse.
- In the case of accumulated pathogenic heat in the intestinal tract: constipation of solid fecal material with watery discharge; fullness, pain, and hard sensation in the abdomen; yellow, thick and dry fur on the tongue; and deep, replete, and forceful pulse.

***Yingfen* Syndrome.** *Yingfen* syndrome shows impaired *ying-yin* (nutritive fluid) due to invasion of *yingfen* by the warm-heat pathogen. This indicates that the morbid condition has developed into a deep and serious stage, clinically characterized by impaired *ying-yin* and mental confusion. Its clinical manifestations are predominant fever at night, slight thirst, vexation, insomnia or coma, delirium, skin rashes, red and crimson tongue, and thready, rapid pulse.

***Xuefen* Syndrome.** This is a critical syndrome indicating invasion of *xuefen* by the warm-heat pathogen. *Xuefen* syndrome is regarded as the last and most serious stage of an epidemic febrile disease. It is clinically characterized by invasion of blood by excessive heat and disorder of mental activities. Clinical manifestations include fever, restlessness, coma, delirium, purple or dark skin eruptions, hemoptysis, epistaxis, hematochezia, convulsion and syncope, reddened or crimson tongue, and thready, rapid pulse. Symptoms may occur as follows:

- In the case of mental disorder due to heat: restlessness, coma and delirium.
- In the case of invasion of blood by excessive heat: skin eruptions, hemoptysis, epistaxis and hematochezia.
- In the case of wind-syndrome due to excessive heat: convulsion and syncope.

If *xuefen* is fumed and scorched by the pathogenic heat: reddened or crimson tongue and small, rapid pulse.

9.10 DIFFERENTIAL DIAGNOSIS IN LIGHT OF THE DOCTRINE OF TRI-*JIAO*

Wu Tang, a distinguished physician of the Qing dynasty, first presented differential diagnosis according to the Doctrine of Tri-*jiao*. He noted that epidemic febrile disease is a general term for all acute febrile diseases caused by different warm-heat pathogens in the four seasons. With seasonal climate changes, the variety exopathogens and the patient's constitution and bodily response, epidemic febrile diseases vary widely in their form, each having its own distinguishing characteristics. In brief, says Wu Tang, doctors can analyze the development of epidemic febrile diseases from the upper part to the lower part of the body and further supplement the differential diagnosis by the analysis of *wei*, *qi*, *ying*, and *xue*.

Damp-heat Syndrome of the Upper-*jiao*. Damp-heat syndrome of the upper-*jiao* is an exterior syndrome due to damp-heat pathogens invading the body at the early stage of an epidemic febrile disease. Since pathogenic dampness is closely related to the spleen and stomach, disturbance of the spleen and stomach due to invasion by pathogenic dampness and its retention in the muscles also appears. The clinical manifestations of this condition are:

- Severe aversion to cold
- Slight fever, no fever, or afternoon fever
- Heavy sensation in the head as if tightly bound and/or heavy sensation in the limbs
- Lassitude
- Chest distension and stuffiness in the epigastrium
- Poor appetite and a sticky taste in the mouth with no feeling of thirst
- Hyponea and borborygmus
- Loose stool
- Whitish and greasy fur on the tongue
- Soft, slow pulse

Damp-heat Syndrome of the Middle-*jiao*. Damp-heat syndrome of the middle-*jiao* is due to damp-heat pathogens invading the body at the middle stage of an epidemic febrile disease, the main pathogenesis of which lies in the retention of the damp-heat pathogen in the spleen and stomach. Its clinical manifestations are:

- Moderate fever that is higher in the afternoon and does not subside after sweating
- Heavy sensation in the limbs
- Lassitude
- Chest stuffiness and abdominal distention
- Nausea and poor appetite
- Thirst with little desire to drink
- Sallow or yellowish complexion
- Hyponea, hypologia, or coma
- Scanty, dark urine, and/or loose stool
- Greyish and yellowish fur on the tongue
- Soft, rapid pulse

The Damp-heat Syndrome of the Lower-*jiao*. Damp-heat syndrome of the lower-*jiao* is due to stagnation of the damp-heat pathogens extending from the middle-*jiao* to the lower-*jiao* in the urinary bladder and the large intestine. This condition leads to dysfunction of the urinary bladder in micturition and the large intestine's functional disturbance. The clinical manifestations of this condition are:

- Dysuria or scanty dark urine
- Thirst with little desire to drink
- Constipation and feeling of hardness and fullness in the lower abdomen or loose stool with tenesmus
- Sensation of distension over the head
- Dizziness
- Greyish, yellowish, and greasy fur on the tongue
- Soft, rapid pulse

CHAPTER 10

Preventative Therapeutic Principles

10.1 OVERVIEW OF PREVENTATIVE THERAPEUTIC PRINCIPLES

Preventative therapeutic principles are those principles that must be followed in the prevention and treatment of disease. TCM has always attached great importance to prevention, and even in *Neijing*, the concept of "preventive treatment of disease" was advanced, stressing "stopping disease before it actually happens."

10.2 PREVENTIVE TREATMENT OF DISEASE

Before the onset of a disease, various preventive measures can be taken to prevent it from occurring. Since the occurrence of a disease involves both the vital *qi* and pathogenic factors, disease prevention must start with enhancing the resistance of vital *qi* to pathogenic factors and with preventing pathogens from invading the body. Therefore, recuperating one's vigor to keep a sound mind, exercising to build up one's health, leading a regular and temperate life, and preventing disease with medicines to build immunity increase body resistance. In addition, developing hygienic habits and preventing pollution of the environment, water supply, and food can also guard against pathogenic invasion.

10.3 CONTROLLING THE DEVELOPMENT OF AN EXISTING DISEASE

Once it occurs, a disease should be diagnosed early and treated and cured in its initial stage, so as to stop it from developing into a more serious state. Moreover, according to the law of disease development, the resistance of the unaffected areas in the human body should be first strengthened. For example, the liver corresponds to wood and the spleen to earth, which is restricted by exuberant wood. That is to say, hyperfunction of the liver (wood) may affect the functioning of the spleen (earth). Therefore, liver disorder is often clinically treated in combination with treatment for strengthening the spleen and stomach in order to make them strong enough to resist liver-pathogens. That is a practical application of the principle regarding controlling the development of an existing disease.

10.4 THERAPEUTIC PRINCIPLES

Therapeutic principles are laws that must be followed in treating disease. Developed under the guidance of wholism and *bianzheng lunzhi* (selection of treatment based on the differential diagnosis), they are also directive rules for guiding establishment of a therapy and prescription of a recipe. Examples include:
- Treatment aimed at the pathogenesis and strengthening of body resistance to eliminate pathogens.
- Regulating *yin* and *yang.*
- Treatment in accordance with seasonal conditions, with local conditions, and with an individual's physique.

10.5 THERAPEUTIC METHODS

The therapeutic methods comprise certain concrete medical treatments, namely, diaphoresis, emisis, purgation, regulation, warming, heat-clearing, invigoration, and resolution. The therapeutic methods are different from the therapeutic principles in that the latter is the general principle guiding the therapeutic method, while the former is the practical application of the therapeutic principle. Any concrete therapeutic method is always based on a definite therapeutic principle. For example, strengthening body resistance to ward off pathogens is a therapeutic principle. On the other hand, invigorating *qi* and *yang* and nourishing the blood and *yin* are concrete methods of strengthening body resistance, and diaphoresis, are concrete methods of eliminating pathogens.

Treatment Aimed at the Primary Cause of Disease. When handling a disease, a doctor must search for its primary cause to adopt a proper treatment. Primary cause of a disease refers to the etiology and pathogenesis of its occurrence and development. Therefore, in treating a disease, a doctor must be adept at finding out its cause and analyzing its pathogenesis in order to treat the disease accordingly. Take headache as an example. It may be caused by attack of exogenous pathogens or internal injury. Headache due to exopathy is of wind-cold type in etiology and, therefore, treatment by relieving the exterior syndrome with drugs pungent in flavor and warm in nature is advisable. On the other hand, the doctor treats a headache due to exopathy of wind-warm type by relieving the exterior syndrome with drugs pungent in flavor and cool in nature. Other headaches may be due to internal injury brought about by different pathogens—such as deficient blood, blood stasis, phlegm-dampness, excessive liver-*yang* and liver-fire—and all would be treated differently.

10.6 ROUTINE TREATMENT

Routine treatment is a commonly used therapeutic principle of treating a disease with the method and drugs contrary to its nature or manifestations. It is suitable when a disease runs according to its nature. Since the manifestations of most diseases coincide with their nature, routine treatment is the most commonly used therapeutic principle. Consequently, treatment of cold syndromes with medicines of hot nature, that of heat syndromes with medicines of cold nature, and that of deficiency syndromes by reinforcement, and that of excess syndromes by purgation are all examples of routine treatment.

Treatment of Cold Syndrome with Hot-natured Drugs. Therapy of cold syndrome with drugs of a hot nature is suitable to interior cold syndrome manifested by cold signs. For example, pain due to direct attack of pathogenic cold on the spleen and stomach manifested as epigastric and abdominal pain may be relieved by warmth and should be treated by warming method to dispel *yin*-cold with drugs pungent in flavor and hot in nature.

Treatment of Heat Syndrome with Cold-natured Drugs. Treating heat syndrome with drugs of a cold nature is suitable to excess-heat type of a febrile-disease manifested by heat signs. For example, symptoms such as high fever, aversion to heat, excessive thirst, profuse sweating and full and large pulse are caused when pathogenic heat (fire) attacks the body. They are treated by clearing the pathogenic heat and purging pathogenic fire with drugs bitter in taste and cold in nature.

Treatment of Deficiency Syndrome by Reinforcement. Treatment of a deficiency syndrome by reinforcement is a therapy for various types of asthenia-syndromes, applicable to a deficiency case that manifests as asthenia-signs. For example, the morbid condition of *yin* deficiency in which *yin* fails to suppress *yang* leads to heat syndrome of deficiency type caused by relative hyperactivity of *yang*. This condition manifests as signs of a deficiency type. Nourishing *yin* to suppress *yang* treats this syndrome. "Restrain *yang* (fire) by nourishing *yin* (water)."

Treatment of Excess Syndrome by Purgation. Purgation is a therapeutic method for treating excess syndromes, applicable to an excess case manifested by excess signs. For instance, retention of pathogenic heat in the stomach and intestines is treated by purgation to remove the retained undigested food in the gastrointestinal tract.

10.7 TREATMENT CONTRARY TO THE ROUTINE

Applying treatment contrary to the routine is a specific therapeutic principle used to treat a disease in accordance with its false signs. That is to say, the nature of drugs prescribed is consistent with its false signs. The false appearances of a disease are phenomena that distort or reverse its nature and are unable to represent its essence. Therefore, when treating a disease, a doctor must see through its appearances to get at its essence. Treatment contrary to the routine appears to conform to the false signs of a disease, but actually it is contrary to its essence. As a consequence, treatments contrary to the routine as well as routine treatments are both practical applications of the therapeutic principle of treating a disease by aiming at its primary causes.

Treatment of Pseudo-heat Syndrome with Hot-natured Drugs. Treating pseudo-heat syndromes with drugs of a hot nature is applicable to treating cold syndrome with pseudo-heat symptoms resulting from *yang* kept externally by *yin*-excess in the interior. For example, *shaoyin* syndrome—characterized by diarrhea with undigested food in stool, cold limbs, feeble and indistinct pulse, but absent of aversion to cold and flushed cheeks—is to a syndrome hot in appearance but cold in nature. Since cold-excess is the essence of the disease, the cold syndrome is treated by a decoction for promoting blood circulation and relieving cold; it is warm or hot in nature, and the pseudo-heat symptoms will disappear by itself.

Treating Pseudo-cold Syndrome with Cold-natured Drugs. Similarly, treating pseudo-cold diseases with drugs of cold nature is applicable to treating heat syndrome with pseudo-cold symptoms, caused by *yin* kept externally by *yang*-excess in the interior. For example, the symptom of cold limbs due to excess of heat marked by cold limbs and deep pulse seems to be cold syndrome, but is accompanied by high fever, feeling of restlessness over the chest, and scanty, dark urine. Since excess heat is the essence of the disease, the heat syndrome must be treated with drugs of cold or cool nature, and subsequently the false manifestations or pseudo-cold symptoms will disappear by themselves.

Treatment of Obstructive Disease with Tonic Drugs. The use of tonic drugs in treating diseases marked by obstructive symptoms is useful when the primary condition is deficiency syndrome with pseudo-excess symptoms such as obstruction syndrome due to the deficiency.

For example, the patient with insufficient spleen usually presents remittent abdominal and epigastric distention, anorexia, pale tongue, and feeble and weak pulse, but in this case does not develop symptoms such as dyspepsia, or stagnation of phlegm-dampness. He or she should be treated with drugs for strengthening the spleen and replenishing *qi*. When spleen-*qi* functions properly in transport, the abdominal distention will subside by itself.

Treatment of Discharging Disease with Purgatives. Purgatives are used as a method of treating excess syndrome when the symptoms indicate excess-syndrome with pseudo-deficiency symptoms. For example, a patient exhibits symptoms, such as diarrhea due to indigestion, metrorrhagia, and metrostaxis due to the retention of stagnated blood in the interior. However, he or she also shows signs of fecal impaction due to heat with watery discharge marked by accumulation of dry feces in the gastrointestinal tract with discharge of foul water. He or she is treated with purgative drugs to eliminate the interior-excess syndrome. Once the interior-excess syndrome is eliminated, the extrinsic discharging symptoms will abate by themselves.

10.8 TREATING A DISEASE BY REMOVING ITS CAUSE OR BY MERELY ALLEVIATING ITS SYMPTOMS

The concept of treating either or both the cause and/or the symptoms represents the fact that any disease has its primary and secondary cause.

- As far as pathogens and vital *qi* are concerned, the latter is primary while the former secondary.
- As far as pathogenesis and symptoms of a disease are concerned, the former is primary whereas the latter secondary.
- As far as the sequence of diseases is concerned, the original or preceding disease is primary while the subsequent disease is secondary.

Frequently, there is a difference between the primary and the secondary causes. In general, in an urgent case, treatment aims at relieving the predominant symptoms (the secondary) first. In a chronic case, however, treatment aims at removing its primary cause. If both the symptoms and the primary cause play an equally important role in the disease's development, treatment should aim at both at the same time.

Relieving the Secondary in an Urgent Case. When the secondary disease is so critical that it becomes the primary contradiction or its primary aspect, it endangers the patient's life or affects the termination of the original disease if not treated promptly. Therefore, emergency measures must be taken to relieve the secondary aspect, to alleviate critical symptoms of a disease, or to relieve the new secondary disease first.

Removing the Primary in a Chronic Case. When the disease becomes alleviated, treatment should aim at the primary disease, which has then become the principal contradiction or its principal aspect. In this case, it is advisable to relieve the primary disease or treat the original disorder according to its cause and pathogenesis. For example, in the case of cough due to pulmonary tuberculosis resulting from *yin* deficient lungs and the kidneys, treatment should aim at removing the primary cause by nourishing *yin* of both the lungs and kidneys. In the case of an old disorder accompanied by a new disease due to exogenous pathogens, which has already subsided, treatment also aims at relieving the primary disease.

Treating the Primary and the Secondary Aspects at the Same Time. When both the primary and secondary diseases are equal in severity and urgency at the same time, treatment should aim at both the primary and the secondary simultaneously. For instance, in the course of a febrile disease, the dryness-heat syndrome cannot be dispelled as a result of profuse consumption of *yin*-fluid, symptoms of deficient vital *qi* and excess of pathogens indicate acute conditions of both the primary and secondary aspects. In this case, *yin*-fluid will be further consumed if one only uses a purgative as treatment; similarly, the dryness-heat cannot be resolved downwards merely by nourishing *yin*. Only by treating the primary and secondary aspects at the same time—that is, only by both nourishing *yin* and purging the dryness-heat to supply fluid—can the aim of eliminating pathogens and supporting vital *qi* be achieved.

Supporting Vital *Qi*. To support vital *qi* is to strengthen body resistance. Since victory or failure in the struggle between vital *qi* and pathogens determines the development or termination of a disease, one of the important principles underlying clinical therapy is to change the relative strength of vital *qi* and pathogens, making the illness take a turn for the better. To support vital *qi* is to restore vital *qi* in most cases, which is indicated when deficient vital *qi* is the primary contradiction and when pathogens are not dominant or have been declining. For example, in the case of deficient *qi*, it is essential to restore *qi*; in the case of deficient *yang*, it is necessary to invigorate *yang*; in the case of deficient *yin*, it is advisable to nourish *yin*; and in ease of blood-deficiency, it is imperative to replenish blood.

Eliminating Pathogens. To eliminate pathogens means getting rid of pathogenic factors to facilitate restoration of vital *qi*. In so doing, pathogens are put off, and vital *qi* is preserved and restored. Therefore, eliminating pathogens, like supporting vital *qi*, is also one of the important principles underlying clinical therapy.

Eliminating pathogens can be achieved mostly by using of purgative methods for excess syndrome when invasion by pathogens is the primary contradiction and vital *qi* has not yet declined. However, the actual therapeutic method employed for this purpose varies greatly with different pathogens and with different sites of their invasion. As examples:

- In the case of attack of the skin by exuberant exogenous pathogens: diaphoretic therapy.
- In the case of invading the upper part of the chest by pathogens accompanied by accumulation of abundant sputum and saliva or prolonged retention of food in the gastrointestinal tract or food poisoning: emetic therapy.
- In the case of invading the lower part of the gastrointestinal tract by pathogens with pathogenic heat combined with waste products in the intestines: purgation.
- In the case of sthenic heat syndrome and sthenic fire-syndrome: heat-clearing and fire-purging therapy.
- In the case of cold syndrome: elimination of pathogenic cold by warming the middle-*jiao.*
- In the case of dampness syndrome: dispelling pathogenic dampness by promoting diuresis.

Supporting Vital *Qi* in Combination with Eliminating Pathogens. This is a therapeutic approach with support of vital *qi* as the dominant factor, supplemented by eliminating pathogens when asthenia-syndrome is accompanied by sthenia-syndrome with the former as the major trouble. By using this approach, pathogens are eliminated and vital *qi* remains unaffected. Instead, the body can be rid of pathogens invading. For example, spleen dysfunction with overabundant dampness is an asthenia-syndrome accompanied with sthenia-syndrome. This condition produces phlegm-dampness in the body and should be treated mainly by invigorating the spleen to support vital *qi*, supplemented by removing phlegm-dampness to eliminate pathogens.

Eliminating Pathogens in Combination with Supporting Vital *Qi*. This is a therapeutic method with elimination of pathogens as the dominant factor, supplemented by support of vital *qi*. It is indicated in sthenia-syndrome accompanied by asthenia-syndrome with excessive pathogens as the main trouble. By using this method, pathogens are generally not to be supported nor retained. Rather, the body's resistance to pathogens can be enhanced. For example, the syndrome of damage of *yin* by hyperactivity of pathogenic heat is a sthenia-syndrome accompanied by sthenia-syndrome with excessive pathogens as the dominant factor. This condition impairs *yin*-fluid in the body due to hyperactivite pathogenic heat and should be treated mainly by eliminating pathogenic heat with the aid of heat-clearing therapy supplemented by support of vital *qi* by nourishing *yin*.

Supporting Vital *Qi* before Eliminating Pathogens. Suitable for asthemia-syndrome accompanied by sthenia-syndrome with deficient vital *qi* as the dominant factor, supporting vital *qi* before eliminating pathogens is viable in cases where vital *qi* in the body is too weak to endure invasion. In this case, if the method of eliminating pathogens is simultaneously applied, vital *qi* will be further damaged instead of being supported. Therefore, supporting vital *qi* before eliminating pathogens is appropriate.

Eliminating Pathogens before Supporting Vital *Qi*. Applicable to sthenia-syndrome accompanied by asthenia-syndrome with excessive pathogens as the dominant factor, eliminating pathogens before supporting vital *qi* is appropriate when vital *qi* in the body is strong enough to resist invading pathogens. In this case, if treatment of supporting vital *qi* is simultaneously applied, pathogens may be encouraged and left in the body. Therefore, eliminating pathogens should be practiced before that of supporting vital *qi* instead of a combination of both at same time.

10.9 REGULATION OF *YIN* AND *YANG*

The relative equilibrium of *yin* and *yang* is restored afresh by regulating their relative strength. The breakdown of *yin-yang* equilibrium is one of the basic pathogeneses of diseases. Therefore, regulating relative strength of *yin* and *yang*, remedying defects, rectifying abuses, and restoring relative equilibrium of *yin* and *yang* constitute one of the most significant principles underlying clinical TCM therapy. Lessening the excess state of *yin* or *yang* while remedying their deficiency is the basic method of regulating *yin* and *yang*.

Lessening the Excess State of *Yin* or *Yang*. Lessening the excess of either *yin* or *yang* applies to sthenic-heat syndrome and sthenic-cold syndrome due to relative excessiveness of *yin* or *yang*. The sthenia-heat syndrome caused by heat due to an excess of *yang* must be treated with drugs of cold or cool nature so as to clear away *yang*-heat. On the other hand, the sthenia-cold syndrome caused by cold due to an excess of *yin* should be treated with hot-natured drugs to warm and expel *yin*-cold.

Further development of relative excessiveness of *yin* or *yang* may lead to deficient either, that is to say, an excess of *yang* leads to disorder of *yin* and vice versa. In the case of sthenic-heat syndrome accompanied by *yin* deficiency resulting from consumption of *yin*-fluid and due to excess of *yang*-heat, heat-clearing therapy in combination with *yin*-nourishing drugs is indicated. In the case of impairment of *yang-qi* due to excess of *yin*-cold, cold-expelling therapy in combination with *yang*-warming drugs is advisable.

Making up for Relative Deficient *Yin* or *Yang*. When asthenic-heat syndrome and asthenic-cold syndrome is caused by relative decline of *yin* or *yang*, it is appropriate to make up for the relative deficient either *yin* or *yang*.

- In the case of asthenic-heat syndrome caused by heat due to *yin* deficiency, treatment should suppress hyperactive *yang* by nourishing *yin*.
- In the case of asthenic-cold syndrome due to *yang* deficiency, treatment should dispel hyperactive *yin* by invigorating *yang*.
- In the case of deficient *yang* affecting *yin*, therapy should invigorate *yang* supplemented by *yin*-nourishing treatment.
- In the case of deficient *yin* affecting *yang*, therapy should invigorate *yin* supplemented by *yang*-nourishing treatment.

10.10 REGULATION OF VISCERAL FUNCTIONS

The human body is an organic whole, in which *zang* organs and *fu* organs coordinate and promote each other physiologically and interact on each other pathologically. When any of the *zang-fu* organs function inadequately, all of the other organs may be affected. Thus, when treating a disorder of any *zang-fu* organ, doctors consider not merely the diseased organ alone, but also the interrelationship between all *zang-fu* organs. For instance, a disorder of the lungs may result either from an attack of pathogens on themselves or from dysfunction of the heart, liver, spleen, kidneys, and the large intestine. Treatments vary as follows:

- In the case of dyspnea and cough due to impaired descending function of lung-*qi* caused by deficient heart-*qi* leading to stagnation of heart-blood: warm heart-*yang* and promote blood circulation.
- In the case of hemoptysis caused by adverse rising of the hyperactive liver-*qi* due to attack of the lungs by the liver-

fire: clear away the liver-fire and send down adversely ascending *qi.*

- In the case of the lung's impaired dispersing and descending functions from production of phlegm due to insufficient spleen and from stagnation of phlegm-dampness in the lungs leading to cough with copious sputum: invigorate the spleen and eliminate pathogenic dampness.

- In the case of dry cough caused by the lungs' consumption of *yin*-fluid, which fail to be nourished due to deficient kidney-*yin*: kidney-nourishing and lung-moistening therapies.

- In the case of dyspnea resulting from adverse ascending of lung-*qi* caused by difficulty in inhalation due to kidney-deficiency: improve inspiration by warming the kidneys.

- In the case of dyspnea caused by dysfunction of lung-*qi* in descent due to retention of pathogenic heat in the large intestine: eliminate sthenia-heat in the large intestine by purgation.

When treating disorders of any *zang-fu* organ, make every effort to regulate the relationship between all *zang-fu* organs, enabling them to coordinate their functions on the basis of the theory of their physiological interconnection and pathological interaction.

10.11 REGULATION OF *QI* AND BLOOD

Qi serves as the commander of blood, which, in turn, acts as the mother of *qi*. When this interaction between *qi* and blood ceases to function appropriately, various disorders ensue. Therefore, when treating a disease, the relationship between *qi* and blood must be regulated to restore their coordination according to the following principle: eliminate what is in excess and make up for what is lacking.

10.12 TREATMENT OF DISEASE IN ACCORDANCE WITH THREE CONDITIONS (SEASONAL CONDITIONS, LOCAL CONDITIONS, AND CONSTITUTION OF AN INDIVIDUAL)

The three conditions form the basis for the therapeutic principle by which an appropriate method of treatment is adopted according to seasonal conditions, local conditions, and physique, sex, and age of an individual. The premise is that various factors—such as climate, geographic-environmental conditions, and an individual's constitutional factors—influence the occurrence, development and termination of a disease in particular. Therefore, in treating a disease, doctors must take into consideration all factors contributing to it to make a concrete analysis of concrete conditions and deal with them in different ways, thereby working out a proper method of treatment.

Treatment in Accordance with Seasonal Conditions. The therapeutic principle underlying the administration of drugs according to climactic variations of different seasons is known as treating of disease in accordance with seasonal conditions. For example, when the climate in late spring and early summer gradually turns from warm to hot, the pores of the body skin are porous. During this time, drastically pungent and warming sudorifics must only be administered with great caution—even in cases of common cold—lest the skin pores open too much and impair *qi-yin*. However, when the climate in late autumn and early winter turns from cool to cold, the pores of the body skin compact and *yang-qi* is full inside the body. At this time, drugs of cold or cool nature should only be administered with great caution—even in cases of febrile disease—lest *yang* should be injured.

Treatment in Accordance with Local Conditions. The therapeutic principle governing administration of drugs according to geographical and environmental features of different localities is called treatment in accordance with local conditions. For example, the common cold in the northwest (severely cold) area is always treated with drastic sudorifics in large doses. In the southeast (warm area), however, it is treated usually with drugs with a milder effect and in smaller doses.

Treatment in Accordance with an Individual's Constitution. The therapeutic principle underlying administration of drugs according to age, sex, physique, and different modes of living is known as treatment in accordance with constitution of an individual. For example, an older person differs from a child not only in age but also in physiological functions and pathological manifestations. Due to deficient *qi* and blood and decline of physiological functions, adults often suffer from deficiency syndrome or asthenia-syndrome accompanied by sthenia-syndrome. In this case, therapy for invigoration is indicated. In the case of excessive pathogens to be eliminated, purgative drugs should be prescribed only with great caution and in doses smaller than those for young people or people during their prime.

Children, who due to exuberant vitality, inadequate *qi* and blood, and delicate and tender *zang-fu* organs, are susceptible to cold or heat, to asthenia or sthenia, may suffer from a disease with a rapid progress. For such a case, therapy for elimination of pathogens should be prescribed only with great caution; tonic therapy is rarely used.

Consideration of these and other personal differences, such as gender, individual physique, etc., take into account the human body as a whole and individual differences among different persons.

Glossary

Abdominal distention

A state in which the abdominal region becomes enlarged or inflated in an abnormal fashion.

Amnesia

A loss of memory.

Anasarca syndrome

Severe generalized edema.

Anxiety

A feeling of apprehension, uneasiness, or dread of the future.

Arthritis

A swelling of a joint usually accompanied by frequent changes in structure.

Banzheng lunzhi

A selection of treatment based on differential diagnosis.

Chong

One of the channels that originates from the uterus.

Cold pathogen

That pathogenic feature which causes cold like disease.

Collateral

A pathway through which qi and blood of the human body are circulated.

Cun

A measurement used for locating acupuncture points. It is the width of the patients thumb.

Da lun

A medical text written by Su Wen.

Dai

One of the eight extra channels.

Damp syndrome

The predominant qi of late summer.

Deficient yang

Situation in the body where yin and yang are not balanced. Patient has more yin than yang qi.

Disease

A pathological condition of the body that presents a group of clinical signs and symptoms that sets the condition apart as an abnormal entity.

Dry Pathogen

Dryness in excess that is disease causing.

Edema

A local or generalized condition in which the body tissues contain an excessive amount of fluid.

Epidemic

The appearance of an infectious disease or condition that attacks many people at the same time.

Epigastrium

Region over the pit of the stomach.

Excess syndrome

That which occurs in the body to remove a situation of balance.

Exopathic factors

Those factors that cause disease which occur outside the body.

Fever
Elevation of body temperature above normal.

Hyperactivity
Increased or excessive activity that may refer to the entire organism or to a particular entity.

Hypoactivity
Decreased activity that may refer to an entire organism or to a particular entity.

Insominia
Inability to sleep at a time when a person expected sleep to occur.

Jaundice
Condition characterized by yellowness of the skin, whites of the eyes, mucous membranes, and body fluids due to deposition of bilirubin in the blood.

Leukorrhea
A white or yellow mucous discharge from the cervical canal or vagina.

Lumbago
A general term for dull aching pain in the lower back.

Miliaria alba
Vesicles caused by obstruction of the ducts of the sweat glands.

Pathogen
Substance capable of producing a disease.

Pathogenesis
Origin and development of a disease.

Phlegm
Thick mucus from respiratory passages.

Viscera
Internal organ enclosed within a cavity.

Index